Overcoming Common Problems

The Heart Recovery Book
A rehabilitation guide

Irene Tubbs

sheldon PRESS

First published in Great Britain in 2006

Sheldon Press
36 Causton Street
London SW1P 4ST

British Library Cataloguing-in-Publication Data
A catalogue record for this book is available from the British Library

ISBN-13: 978–0–85969–955–6
ISBN-10: 0–85969–955–2

1 3 5 7 9 10 8 6 4 2

Typeset by Avocet Typeset, Chilton, Aylesbury, Bucks
Printed in Great Britain by Ashford Colour Press

Contents

Acknowledgements

In essence we're all 'helpers', thriving and learning from our own and others' life experiences, and in turn sharing what we have learnt. I am indebted to all the past and present members of my coronary rehab groups for their support in sharing such experiences. In particular, their tenacity in dealing with their heart condition and its consequent stresses enabled me to add to my own 'self help' strategies and to develop my professional beliefs in such a way that I could devise processes for change that are achievable stratagems for improved health and wellbeing.

Introduction

Our health is central – evident when we greet someone with 'How are you?' and saying, as they leave, 'Take care'. Yet many of us take our health for granted until illness develops. In this book I'm seeking to talk to you as someone I have met many times, someone who may still be in shock, pain, disbelief, perhaps thinking, 'How did I get this condition?' or, with some relief, 'At last I've been sorted out'. You may still be fearful of the future and your ability to support both yourself and any medical treatments.

So who am I? I'm Irene, and I have worked within community-based coronary rehabilitation for over 25 years. When I was first a young physical education specialist, all that time ago, I was approached by the Inner London Education Authority to run community-based exercise classes in partnership with Dr M. A. Scott, Consultant Physician at Lewisham hospital, who had established hospital-based rehab courses.

People (just like you) requested help with continuation of exercise after they had completed the course, in order to remain healthy in the future. I soon realized they wanted to develop a personalized programme of fitness, and that is where it all began. Then, as now, they were wanting to help themselves, as I am sure you are.

Working with people who had experienced heart conditions such as high blood pressure, heart attack, marfan syndrome, valve replacement, by-pass surgery, heart transplant, or had been treated for irregular heartbeats, angina and stroke, I developed these exercise-based programmes into a holistic format that included many other lifestyle factors.

At the request of a great number of people, and also the many people I visited on the wards, I gathered together a wide variety of complementary self-help strategies into my book *Put Your Heart Into It – self-help guidelines for anyone who has a condition that affects the heart* (1990), which was published by the Adult Education Institute for local coronary rehab patients (although many copies ended up in Malta!). It has been very interesting reviewing this past work, which was last updated in 1994, as the majority of its content is still relevant today.

Yet although there have been extensive changes in palliative care since then, there are still inconsistencies relating to recovery guidelines. My recent study of 110 people (2005) highlighted these continuing inconsistencies, with similar comments made to those I received 15 years ago. So what's missing?

While there are copious medical books and leaflets relating to heart conditions and excellent information booklets from the British Heart Foundation (BHF), people differ in their ability to process the information. They need a format that puts everything under one banner, is easy to access, and is readable – but, most importantly, that encourages them to be proactive in their own recovery. They need written information that not only gives guidelines on the prevention of another bout of their illness, but recognizes the diversity of individual experiences of illness. I have sought to ensure this in *The Heart Recovery Book* by listening to those who have suffered, ascertaining how much they do know and wish to know, and compiling this into progressive programmes that do not insist on unrealistic gains or instant changes, but work within a time frame that is feasible for each individual.

This book suggests many different ways to deal with and support recovery after heart attack, heart disease, heart surgery or other procedures, using constructive ways to feel in control *of*, instead of controlled *by*, your illness. It is not, however, intended as a substitute for the advice of your GP, dietician or cardiologist, but instead is a complementary recovery tool.

Some of you will still be awaiting medical appointments and/or treatments, and while you wait, you can use this 'self-help' book to review constructive coping strategies and use them before you go into hospital.

Most importantly, remember that the body is a wonderful complex, self-generating healer that will seek to repair itself once an identified problem has arisen, supported by you adopting and practising healthy habits alongside the use of prescribed medications and/or surgery.

Over the years I have seen many coronary rehab patients make such changes in their lives that they actually feel healthier after their condition surfaced than they did before. You can do it too. Practice is the key to maintaining effective change. Use this book and others to support you. Start today!

1

Towards improved health

Let's begin as we mean to go on, with the good news: deaths from heart disease are falling.

A Department of Health report (2004) stated, 'New advances in treatments continue to develop and, linked with changes in lifestyles, have resulted in the number of 65-year-olds dying from heart disease falling from 90 men and 25 women per 10,000 in 1990 to 50 men and 10 women in every 10,000 in 2000.'

Evidence of such improvement can be seen with the following two examples:

John

Before diagnosis, John was a 61-year-old who ate a lot of cakes, pies, biscuits and sweets, only drank one glass of wine a day, but had smoked all his life, and although he did a manual job he recognized he wasn't doing enough exercise. The first indicator of something being wrong was chest pain.

After diagnosis of a heart attack, and being prescribed medication, John has changed his diet, increased his level of exercise, and socializes more, particularly with those with the same condition. John says, 'Although I'm still suffering with occasional night sweats and cramps, I feel happier, more content, more relaxed and pleased with my life.'

Anne

Before diagnosis, Anne was a 56-year-old who often got easily agitated, leading to angry outbursts. She also suffered with extreme fatigue and increasing bouts of breathlessness.

After diagnosis of blocked arteries, and undergoing by-pass surgery, she still gets agitated but not so intensely, and feels more motivated and optimistic about life, particularly since developing an exercise regime.

As you can see, one of the people just mentioned had noticed warning signals, and the other had not. Sometimes a heart attack can have occurred, but the person may not realize it until after they have had further tests. The relevance of this is crucial to your recovery because it is so easy to become oblivious to our body's messages: occasional pains in the chest or aches down the arms, or even being a bit overtired or breathless. These symptoms are frequently put down to eating too fast, rushing or overworking.

The essence of this book is secondary prevention through various life changes, but most importantly through listening to your body and its messages in order to deal with any difficulty before it reaches a point of major discomfort or illness. I hasten to add here that this does not mean that you should keep listening to your heartbeat – in fact, quite the opposite. Don't!

We begin our programme of health changes by reviewing what you probably felt like before or while you were in hospital. Here are some examples from rehab participants – do you recognize any of these feelings? If the answer is yes, then you're normal!

- Numbness and shock, e.g. 'Never been ill before'.
- Fear of more pain or disability, e.g. 'Will I be an invalid now?'
- Anxiety, isolation and insecurity, e.g. 'I can't cope/don't understand why'.
- Loss of identity, e.g. 'Who am I? Who will I be now?'
- Fear of nearness of death, e.g. 'Should I make a will?'
- Relief, e.g. 'It wasn't just stress causing my hypertension'.
- Anxiety about the future, e.g. 'What warning signs do I look for in the future?'
- Worries concerning prevention of further illness, e.g. 'What can I do to stop it happening again?'

Family reactions, real or imagined, can also be a source of distress – you may fear they can't cope with your illness, find it too upsetting, pity you or, conversely, insist that everything is all right. You may say little to them for fear of upsetting them further, though some people find that telling the family how you feel removes a lot of pressure. Asking others for help can sometimes be a problem too.

What do you think your family's anxieties were or are now? Here are some examples of the reaction of relatives:

- Shock, 'It can't be'.
- Fear, 'Will they die?'
- Anger, 'Why didn't you tell me how you were feeling?'
- Anxiety, 'How will they cope with it?'

- Guilt, 'Why didn't I see it was happening and make them see the doctor?'
- Inadequacy, 'How am I going to cope with so much else to do?'
- Pressure demands, 'I must look after them, stop them from making things worse'.
- Financial worries, 'What will we do for money?'
- Employment worries, 'Can they return to work?'
- Communication difficulties, 'What can I do to help them and get them to listen to me?'
- Isolation, 'I feel so alone; I want others to help me, but I'm afraid to ask'.
- Confusion, 'They're the experts – they should sort the problems out'.
- Keeping up a front, 'I've got to put on a brave face and not show any concern in front of her'.

All the above fears are normal – in fact, if you are the person with the heart condition or his or her relative, and were not feeling some of them before, during or after treatment, I would be concerned! Some of these emotions and fears were probably released and relieved by the support you received in hospital. For those still awaiting hospital admission, use the following section to understand what to expect.

Medical advice – in hospital

When you first entered hospital, a team of specialist cardiac nurses and doctors treated you, and you were dependent on their expertise (and probably watching their every word and movement). Your role was to stay as calm as possible and respond to their questions.

You probably felt fear and anxiety, but also had some security and peace of mind in knowing that you were in an environment that would be able to respond to your needs. It is therefore understandable that we sometimes tend to expect others with specialist skills to make all the decisions and simply tell us what to do.

Yet even the hospital regime requires people to take an active part in their recovery. For example, you had to voice any concerns or fears and ask for help, and listen to and write down any advice, such as:

- After angioplasty, lie still for several hours.
- After surgery, report any signs of infection of the wound to the doctor immediately; keep chest and leg scars dry; use unscented soaps and no bath lotions or softeners when washing; discuss with the physiotherapist and the rest of the medical team how much, and what type of, physical activity is suitable for you.
- Begin exercise regimes including walking up and down the ward, climbing stairs, neck and circulation exercises, and deep breathing.
- Get out of bed, sit at the table and eat with others.
- Use distraction techniques (such as coughing) to deal with injections.
- Start taking medication and use the opportunity to ask what it is for.
- Put into practice your recovery guidelines (more of this below).

Recovery advice

Advice is the primary support tool for people, but over the years, according to coronary rehab patients in my own classes, this has varied from nothing at all to extensive information, either from the coronary unit, the British Heart Foundation (BHF) or local GPs. So, if your recovery advice was less than satisfactory, you will probably benefit from reading the guidelines and information below.

While they mainly deal with issues for people recovering from surgery, they will also be of benefit to anyone who has a condition that affects the heart.

Post-surgery symptoms

There are certain general symptoms you may have experienced after surgery that may cause some anxiety. These symptoms are usually nothing to worry about, and are only part of the surgical trauma and the healing process that follows, but always inform your doctor as soon as possible if you are concerned. They are:

- *Tingling in the fingers* – this is not angina returning, but part of the trauma of surgery. It may take some months to pass.
- *Weird dreams* or seeing things that you cannot really relate to

(illusions or hallucinations). The reason for this distressing symptom is that during surgery you were put on a special machine, which enabled the blood to circulate your body while the operation was in progress, but by-passed the heart so that surgery could take place. Don't be alarmed, such dreams will pass in time. When waking up, use your imagination to change them into positive endings.

- *Pain near your chest or leg incision* will continue to be a nuisance for a few weeks. Continue taking your painkillers, even if only first thing in the morning to help you start the day, and last thing at night to help you to rest. Have frequent baths.
- *Redness, soreness or discharge from your wounds and fever* – if you notice any of these, go to your GP as soon as possible. If you have a leg wound and the leg looks swollen, continue with your walking programme to improve the circulation and reduce the swelling. When sitting, support your legs so that they are slightly raised above your bottom (a pillow under the feet and knees is helpful) and circle each ankle four times each way every hour.
- *Moods (post-op blues)* – you may have the odd day when you feel very low and disinclined to do anything. This is common after surgery. Just let the day drift by and share your feelings with someone else.
- *Constipation* can occur after any stay in hospital, due to lack of exercise, anxiety, drugs, pain from surgery and change of diet. Eat more fruit, e.g. prunes; eat more fibre, e.g. bran; continue to exercise. Drink a cup of hot water first thing in the morning. If constipation persists, tell your doctor.
- *Problems lifting objects* – do not lift too much in the early stages of your recovery, especially if you have undergone surgery. A good guideline is not to carry any weights over 4 pounds (equivalent to two bags of sugar), including children. Shop more frequently, buy smaller amounts, or purchase a trolley (do not overload it).
- *Angina, breathlessness, tiredness or swollen ankles* – if you suffer from any of these, always consult your GP as soon as possible.
- *Common infections* can play a part in triggering acute heart and circulatory problems, so you need to be careful. At the first sign of a cold, or a sense of feeling unwell, go to your GP as soon as possible as the risks increase in the first three days of

an illness, when you are susceptible to developing respiratory tract infections such as bronchitis or pneumonia, or other conditions such as cystitis. If you do become unwell, even if it is only a cold, ensure you keep warm. Wear several layers of light clothing, so that if you become overheated you can just take one off. Eat a good diet and, if possible, ensure that in the future you have a flu jab. Otherwise, be alert and listen to your body.
- *Any dental problems* – anyone with a heart condition needs to pay special attention to the state of their teeth, but especially if they have undergone valve surgery (read the section on dental hygiene in Chapter 2).

Other areas of concern

Other immediate issues for people recovering from surgery or other heart procedures or heart conditions are smoking and drinking, driving, holidays and travel, sex, and work:

Smoking and drinking

You should of course have given up smoking (if not, read Chapter 9); alcohol in moderation can be good for you. If you are on warfarin therapy, this advice concerning alcohol still applies, but you must be especially careful *never* to binge-drink, as this alters clotting factors and makes estimation (where your blood is tested) difficult. (Read Chapter 10 for more on alcohol.)

Driving

If you have a straightforward recovery after a heart attack, you will be able to start driving again after four weeks. If you feel anxious and suffer with angina, use your spray under the tongue before you drive. The breathing technique I will show you later (see Chapter 5) reduces anxiety, and so lessens the likelihood of an angina attack. If you do suffer an angina attack while driving, stop immediately, and wait until you recover, or call for help, before driving on.

If you have undergone surgery, do not drive until you have attended your first outpatients appointment (usually about six weeks after discharge) and been cleared by your GP. People having valve surgery must inform the Driver and Vehicle Licensing Agency (DVLA). Those having grafts need not, but do let your insurance company know in case your condition affects your cover. If you have a licence to drive a large goods vehicle (LV) or a passenger-carrying vehicle (PCV), you must let the DVLA know about your heart attack or surgery. You will undoubtedly be asked to undertake a number of tests before a decision is made about whether you can keep your licence.

Holidays

Spending time with your loved ones is a good idea, but holidaying abroad is not advisable until you have seen your cardiac surgeon at outpatients. If you really wish to fly, the guideline is: 'If you can walk 100 yards on the flat briskly and without chest pain or too much breathlessness, you are fit to travel by air', but always check with your GP first. If you have a pacemaker, tell the airport staff, so that you by-pass any security systems that could affect it. If while flying you get angina, it is safe to use your GTN spray in a pressurized container while on the plane. If you have difficulty with obtaining travel insurance cover, the BHF have a list of companies that are sympathetic to those with heart problems. On the plane, practise the circulation and sitting exercise programmes detailed in Chapter 13.

Physical intimacy

It is understandable that sex may be an area of concern. To feel wanted and to want someone else is a natural comforter, and in the initial stages of recovery it is important for many to be able to enjoy frequent cuddles and massage. Sex itself does increase the heart rate and blood pressure, and some people with heart disease may initially experience breathlessness or chest pain. However, all my clients feel this is more due to anxiety (which leads to surges of adrenaline that make the heart beat faster) rather than sex itself.

The BHF recommendation is that if you have a heart attack, you can safely start having sex again two or three weeks after the attack. If you are concerned, or if you are suffering impotence, talk to your GP.

If, however, you tend to have angina attacks brought on by physical exertion you should:

- Avoid sex within two hours of a heavy meal.
- Keep the bedroom warm and avoid cold sheets, and ensure the atmosphere is relaxing.
- Avoid alcohol for at least three hours before sex.

- Avoid sex if you are tense and tired.
- Get into a comfortable position (passive initially).
- Take your GTN medicine beforehand, keeping it at the bedside just in case you need it.

Sex can usually be safely enjoyed three to four weeks after surgery, provided you've made a good recovery. However, bear in mind that after-effects of an operation, such as the chest scar, may cause pain or discomfort.

Find a position that is comfortable for you and your partner, one that will not stress your chest wound or restrict your breathing, and adopt a passive role initially. Cuddling during the first four weeks helps you to relax and relieves anxiety. It is usually safe to have sex if you can walk about 300 metres on the level comfortably, or climb two flights of stairs briskly without getting chest pains or becoming breathless. (Follow my advice on exercise in Chapter 13 and you'll soon be there.)

Some medicines, such as regular beta-blockers and calcium antagonists, increase the amount of exercise or activity you can do and can help relieve symptoms that can be brought on by sex.

Returning to work

Returning to work can be a viable and motivating option and this can happen as early as six weeks after a heart attack, particularly where the workload is light.

However, if your job requires effort, or if you have undergone surgery, at least three months is needed for bones, muscles and the joints of the chest wall to heal before you return to work. Talk to your GP, your consultant and your employers. Many firms are accommodating to the needs of their employees; after all, when you don't work, they lose an asset. See if your employer is willing to allow you perhaps a staggered start, until you feel ready to resume full time. Some people I know have gone back on a reduced-hours basis, which they prefer to full days. Or, if your job has been stressful, now could be the time to consider a change or early retirement.

Fear of losing your job is common during early recovery. On the rare occasion that firms are not accommodating, it should be realized that the Disability Discrimination Act highlights that employers cannot discriminate against employees because of a declared disability. Your illness therefore cannot be a condition for dismissal or redundancy unless your employers can show that it would be unreasonable to make modifications necessary to allow a disabled person to do a specific job.

However, although you will probably have been given some excellent information from the BHF on your condition and ways to cope, you may need some extra help and support, so contact the BHF (see Useful Addresses) as they have over 180 nurses with different roles and remits who can advise you.

By putting the above suggestions into practice, you begin the process of feeling in control of, instead of controlled by, your condition – which is the most essential element of any recovery from illness. If, however, you experience any symptoms that are not listed here and they worry you, go to your GP as soon as possible.

When you are discharged from hospital

It is natural to feel a mixture of positive and negative emotions when you are discharged from hospital: relief, happiness to be returning home, but also fear as to whether you'll be able to cope or go back to work, whether the surgery has been successful, and whether you are able to manage any fatigue or pain, cope with people or feel irritable, or simply want to retreat into your shell. Undoubtedly you will want to return to your normal way of life, yet this may still seem a long way off.

Statistics suggest that as many as 30 per cent of people report feeling anxious or depressed after a heart attack or heart surgery. In my experience, the figures are much higher. How can you not be anxious or fearful when you have had such a shock? These are perfectly normal reactions, but if left to fester they will increase anxiety and stress levels which will slow down the recovery process.

Be confident that you would not have been discharged from hospital unless you were considered fit to go home.

On leaving hospital you need to take with you:

- Medication and a written list of what it is for, when to take it, and for how long.
- Discharge letter and details of any prescriptions to be given to your own GP.
- Leaflets explaining your condition and advice for your recovery.

- Written-down answers from medical staff to questions you have asked.
- Someone to accompany you home (or someone at home to meet and stay with you for at least some part of the first few days if you live alone).
- Follow-up appointment date.

2

Back home – some practicalities

This is where the real self-help journey begins!

Carers and loved ones will have a natural desire to wrap you up in cotton wool, and you may relish a bit of tender loving care at first, and maybe at intervals later on too. Time is also undoubtedly a healer, but instead of sitting and waiting for your body to do its work, you can help the process along by a progressive programme of movement (see Chapter 13).

Although you will naturally tire easily in the early stages of recovery, this is just your body encouraging you to take it easy. By all means listen to it, but remember, just like a battery, your body needs constant charging to keep it in tip-top condition. Leave it idle and its efficiency depletes.

Your road to recovery may be up and down, but if you believe in your ability to make changes and put into practice the suggestions within this book, you will be able to live your life to the full.

Hopefully you will have been contacted by a rehabilitation nurse before you left hospital and been given information on coronary rehabilitation programmes (details of such programmes can be found on page 98).

Meanwhile, this chapter looks at the practical aspects of your daily life that you're likely to face when you return home.

Medication

You will have been prescribed either singularly, or as a combination, the following medications to support your body on its road to recovery and to act as secondary prevention barriers. These prescription drugs are designed to:

- Balance out high or low blood pressure.
- Lower cholesterol.
- Deal with angina attacks (spray or tablet).
- Disperse and thin blood that is overly clotting, thereby improving circulation.
- Encourage a regular heart rhythm.

- Reduce water retention.
- Relieve breathlessness and the likelihood of heart failure.

DO:

- Take your pills as prescribed.
- Report any side effects.
- Take enough pills with you when you are travelling.
- Check with the pharmacist or your doctor if the dispensed tablets appear to have changed in shape or colour from your previous prescription.
- Consult your GP before you take any homeopathic remedies.
- Avoid eating grapefruit or drinking grapefruit juice if you are taking cholesterol-lowering drugs.

DO NOT:

- Forget to take your pills.
- Run out of pills.
- Start any other medication (including cold remedies) without consulting your doctor.
- Miss appointments with your GP.
- Stop taking your medication if you experience side effects without first consulting your doctor.
- Take other people's pills because they seem to have the same complaint and their tablets work for them – not everyone is the same.

Warfarin

If you have been prescribed warfarin, you will have been given a card and a booklet. Carry it with you at all times. Here is a reminder of the important do's and don't's of warfarin therapy.

DO:

- Always take as prescribed.
- Take at the same time each day.
- Keep appointments for blood checks.
- Inform your dentist and GP that you are taking warfarin.
- Notify your GP if you bruise or bleed abnormally.

DO NOT:

- Take aspirin or drugs containing aspirin (this will thin your blood further).
- Take any other medication, including vitamins, without first consulting your GP.
- Drink excessive alcohol, although a daily drink is safe.
- Drink cranberry juice if you are on warfarin.

Stress-reducing tools to cope with medication

Some people have several medications to take, creating anxiety as to how much, when, how frequently and for how long to take them. There are several coping options:

1 As soon as you return home from the pharmacist, write on each container exactly what your pills are for, e.g. fluid retention, heart, arthritis, sleeping tablet, how many and when to take them. This will also be useful for other family members, especially if they have to administer your medicine. Sometimes the prescribed dosage is higher than that actually manufactured or supplies are low, so that you have to take more than one tablet. Make sure you write on the bottle the number of pills you need to take.

2 You can buy a small hand-held pill container that has compartments clearly marked and separated into breakfast, lunch, teatime and bedtime sections for each medication for each day. Once a week, these compartments are filled. These are easily checkable on your chart and safe for a week, as you only slide the plastic top back to release the tablets for that day. These containers are available from the London Association for Blind People (see Useful addresses) and many chemists. The Royal National Institute for the Blind also support the use of 'talking labels' on medication containers which, when pressed, tell you the correct dosage to take.

3 Keep a chart inside the medicine cabinet door detailing what needs to be taken and when. An example is given in Table 2.1.

Table 2.1 An example of a medication chart to keep inside the medicine cabinet

Medication	*How many pills to take*	*How often*	*For how long*
Aspirin	One tablet	Daily – mornings	Indefinitely
Warfarin	Two tablets	Daily – mornings	Indefinitely
Cholesterol-reducer	One tablet	Daily – mornings	Until cholesterol is down
Blood pressure	One tablet	Daily – mornings	Until told otherwise
Angina spray	Two puffs	When required	Indefinitely

Medication and your GP

It is imperative that you contact or visit your GP a week before your tablets run out for a repeat prescription. A face-to-face consultation is more reassuring than re-ordering over the phone, especially as you can tell your GP of any discomfort or side effects you have experienced on the medication. Also, report any physical sensations you are experiencing, no matter how trivial they may seem.

Getting medication right is obviously essential for everyone, but it is important that you take an active part in such selection. While I am not suggesting you constantly scrutinize papers or articles on new drugs, do keep an eye out and, where appropriate, take the article along to your GP and ask about it.

Regular monitoring by your GP of your blood pressure, height and weight, and tests for cholesterol levels, are all essential. But you should wait six weeks after a heart attack or surgery before having your cholesterol read as you can have a false reading. When blood cholesterol levels have been checked, after due consideration of other risk factors, drugs known as ‘statins’ can be prescribed. They have been found to significantly reduce the risk of strokes and glaucoma and help prevent deep vein thrombosis, osteoporosis and breast cancer and arthritis symptoms in 31 per cent of people.

Dental hygiene

Always tell your dentist of your condition, so that if necessary antibiotic cover can be given before treatment begins.

Research in 2004 (Columbia University, New York) showed that poor dental hygiene not only leads to bad breath and gum disease, but increased susceptibility to developing narrowing of the arteries that can cause heart attacks and strokes. Because once bacteria gets into the bloodstream, they lead to inflammation that results in clogging and, in some cases, an infection of the heart lining (endocarditis).

Daily flossing is vital for healthy teeth and gums as it prevents the build-up of bacteria. Ensure teeth are kept clean and have regular dental check-ups. Tell your cardiologist and your GP of any dental problems whenever you visit them. Some doctors will prescribe medication (usually antibiotics) if you are to have further surgery, so that any bacteria is dealt with before your operation.

Seeing your doctor again

This is unavoidable at some point, but can be a source of distress to many, particularly if, as is quite common, you feel you're being processed through the medical machine rather than really being listened to.

Do have a look at the other chapters in this book, particularly Chapter 5, which show you techniques to help you face this situation more calmly. Meanwhile, let's look at how preparation and effective communication skills helped in the case of Ron, who came to one of my classes:

Ron

Ron needed to visit the consultant to find out about his condition and treatment. Previous visits had led to him feeling frustrated – and in one case he'd had an angry outburst – because he felt he was not being listened to. Before the visit he slept badly, experienced anxiety, tightness in the chest, and greater stiffness and pain in his legs. He also had negative thoughts, such as 'I bet it'll be like last time, he never listens to me. I bet there's something really wrong and he's afraid to say so, in case I lose my temper again.' Or, 'What have I done to deserve this pain, it's not fair, why me? It's because I'm no one special – they wouldn't treat me like this if I could pay. What's the point of going?' He was also ratty with his wife and consequently distressed.

I explored with Ron not only what caused the anxiety, but also the benefits of practising effective communication skills. First, I reviewed body language, the way he sat, the importance of eye contact, the position of the chair he was sitting on, and so on.

Ron rehearsed his doctor's appointment with me, using deep breathing and other techniques to feel back in control. He particularly liked the idea of eye contact and the placement of the chair, saying, 'You know, he always sits me to one side, but now I'm going to move the chair.' This is what Ron reported after his appointment:

> The doctor started to talk before I had even sat down, so I said, 'Just give me a minute to sit down please, I want to make sure I hear you.' He apologized, which really surprised me, and I was able to admit to him that I got nervous and that he talked too fast, and he then promised to slow down. I then asked him my questions (he had to tell *me* to slow down!), making sure I looked him in the eye. Do you know, that was the first time I felt listened to. I could see he was being honest. I realized that a lot of the past relationship problems was me, I was just so scared he was going to tell me that he couldn't help me. I'm always going to write my questions down from now on and breathe when I feel frustrated.

We need to check out the unspoken messages we believe are being relayed by others. There is no doubt that some people 'read' messages from medical practitioners that are not helpful, but do not question these. I once had a scan when the radiologist was continually shrugging her shoulders and sighing. After some anxiety I asked what was wrong. She replied, 'Nothing, I always do that when I'm concentrating.' How many people would ask? Not many in my experience – they tend to become distressed and 'awfulize'.

Ron explored the following suggestions at home before visiting his doctor. You can try them too:

- If you are going to the doctor on your own, practise beforehand by placing a chair so that it is straight and opposite another chair (preferably with a table in between). Ensure when you sit down that your position enables you to be in eye contact with the opposite chair. Also check that your own back rests firmly against the back of the chair and sit comfortably, arms uncrossed (resting on the arms of the chair is best).
- If you are going to the doctor with your partner, put two chairs side by side facing forwards, and sit on them, with one chair opposite you both. You will see that the control would be with the medical

practitioner, who can easily focus on only one person. Now get up and slightly move both your chair and your partner's so that they are angled towards each other, almost touching at one corner at the front and giving a ^ shape at the back. Such a position enables you to easily seek the support of your partner if needed, and ensures that the medical practitioner speaks to both of you.

- Write down all the questions you want answered no matter how trivial they may seem and then try to condense them into five. If you are attending with your partner or carer, or if you are going on your own, discuss the questions with someone before you go. For example, with regard to your medication, ask:

  What is the drug's name?
  How will it affect my condition?
  When and how often should I take it?
  How much should I take each time?
  What are the possible side effects?
  Would I be able to increase/decrease the dose without consulting you?
  Should I avoid taking other non-prescribed medication, e.g. cold remedies or alcohol, while on this drug?
  Is this drug addictive, and will I have to take it for ever?
  How long will it be before the drugs start to take effect and I feel better?

  Also, take with you written notes of any difficulties you have been experiencing with your condition.

When you go for your outpatients appointment

- Take a book, magazine or paper to distract you from focusing on the clock or your watch while you are waiting to be seen. Ask when you book in if there is any additional waiting time, e.g. if the clinic is running late. If it is going to be a very long wait, instead of just sitting there, go and have a cup of tea or have a short walk; or if you are worried about not finding (or losing) a seat, take a flask of tea or a cold drink with you.
- If you start to feel agitated, remember to take a deep breath and think, 'It's annoying to have to wait, but I *will* be seen and that's what is important.'

- Before you enter the room, take two deep breaths – the last one as you actually enter. Make sure you have your list of questions and a pen to write down the answers.
- As you enter the room, look at the placement of the chairs and make sure you move them to a position that is comfortable for you, even if it's only a few inches. Take a deep breath and sit down.
- Look the doctor in the eye when he or she speaks to you. It is likely that they will begin by asking you how you have been, and this is the time to read from your notes. After listening to the medical information, take out your question list and, as you do so, take a deep breath, look at them and say, 'I have a few questions I would like to ask you before I leave' and write down the answers as you hear them. (See Chapter 5 for more on breathing techniques for potentially stressful situations.)

Your environment

Many people feel extremely depressed by the conditions in which they live, and this can certainly worsen during and just after your illness. For some who work, being at home, while initially comforting, can be worrying in terms of chores and tasks that need doing. For specific techniques to tackle distress, and to help you arrange your priorities, look at the 'ABCDE' process in Chapter 8; meanwhile, consider the following:

- Accept your recovery will take time, which will naturally create limitations. Let others help you; you will be helping them by relieving their worries about you 'overdoing it'. Ask family and friends or neighbours to help with repairs that need a lot of effort and tend to bring on angina attacks.
- If you can afford it, allow other professionals to do jobs in the home.
- If you are determined to do the tasks yourself, break them down into manageable chunks. Work out your best time of day and only do the absolutely essential element of that task for that day. During the first three months, never work more than one to two hours at any one time. You need to rest to recoup that energy. Working when you are tired leads to fatigue and stress, so the finished results may not be to your usual standard.

- If money problems stop you doing decorating, a good spring-clean will often revive a room or just touch up the bits you really feel need it. Remember it is your home, and your comfort is all you need to worry about. Outsiders rarely notice what you feel needs decorating; they have come to visit you, not view your house.
- Confrontation with neighbours can be a major stress for some people. Try to talk through any problems calmly with your neighbour. If this is not working, avoid the situation for now, or talk to someone who can advise you. Neighbourhood Watch schemes can alleviate the stress of being lonely or the fear of being burgled, providing support and contact with your neighbours. There are also many local agencies that you can turn to for help, such as the Citizens Advice Bureau, the council's Environmental Health department, and Age Concern.
- The walking programme is particularly helpful to those who are afraid to leave their homes after illness (see Chapter 13) and can help you see your environment in a different light, but always walk during the day and preferably with someone.

Sleeping difficulties

Sleeping difficulties are increasing, with three out of ten of us suffering at least once a week, and this may affect your recovery. Factors that make it worse are our 24-hour society, laptop computers in bedrooms, phones, light and noise pollution, worry, your partner snoring, and the belief that 'I never get enough sleep'.

While sleep is essential, the amount we actually need depends on our age and the way we live our lives. When we are recovering from illness, frequent naps are restorative. Scientific studies have confirmed that a nap is good for our health because after 30 minutes' sleep, growth hormones are released into the body, stimulating the natural repair and growth of muscle tissue. Yet some people stop themselves from napping for fear of not being able to sleep at night, which often leads to over-tiredness as well as a greater difficulty in going to sleep.

First, set the scene for restful and refreshing sleep:

- Ensure your curtains are sufficiently thick to cut out the light, even in the daytime. Initially, in the early stages of recovery, lie down on your bed rather than sleep in a chair, as this is the better recovery posture.

- Turn any clock away from you. Digital lights or even ticking can disturb sleep.
- Have several lightweight covers, not tucked in, for ease of movement.
- If you wake up after a few hours, instead of looking at the time and thinking, 'Oh, no, I've only had three hours' sleep' (a negative upsetting thought), try to think, 'Oh good, at least I've had three hours' sleep' (a realistic and positive thought).
- An open window for ventilation often aids sleep as fresh air is a wonderful relaxant, but it depends on your home situation. Sometimes this allows noise into the room or creates a draught. If this is the case, have the window open before you go to bed, and close it once you get into bed.
- Sleep encourages the release of leptin, which helps suppress the production of fat cells by curbing the appetite. But eating close to going to bed means that the body does not have time to digest the food and therefore stores the material as fats, inhibiting sleep because you feel so full. Try to have at least three hours' 'digestion' time before you go to bed.

If you are still unable to sleep

Have a pen and paper by the side of your bed. If you have worries about jobs that need doing, write them down so you have a reminder to do them tomorrow.

If the thoughts stem from anxiety, anger, frustration and so on, write down the thoughts exactly as you think them, read the list once only, and then tear up the paper into tiny pieces and think 'That's that rubbish out'.

If the thoughts persist, try this distraction technique. Just one word of caution – if you have problems with your eyes or you feel uncomfortable when you try this, do not continue to do so. Just do the deep breathing instead.

- Close your eyes and feel your pupils move up and down and side to side. Repeat four times.
- Open your eyes and try to look into the back of your eyelids (this tires the eyes) and count to ten.
- Slowly lower the eyelids until they close, counting to ten.
- Repeat both processes twice more.

- Take four deep breaths and feel your whole body soften and, if you can, roll on to your side, in what is known as the recovery position. (For more on relaxing breathing techniques, see Chapter 14.)
- In Chapter 14 I will demonstrate a full relaxation process that many of the people in my own classes use to go to sleep at night. Apparently my voice sends them off!

Soreness and sleep

If you have a sore chest from an operation scar and need to lie on your back, it can be difficult to go to sleep. Many people initially experience this problem, but most say that with time they get used to it. But for those who didn't, we found ways to help them.

One lady found her scar tissue particularly sore and very painful in the night. Whenever she rolled over, it would wake her up. We made a soft cotton chest pad, filled with cotton wool for both her back and chest, held by cotton straps and Velcro tape, so that when she rolled over she was not awoken by sudden pain. She phoned me to say, 'I slept last night for the first time without waking. I was so relieved I cried this morning.' Another man found that a steroid cream given to him by his doctor eased the soreness.

Remember, if you are woken up by pain, you will automatically hold your breath, which increases the pain. Encourage yourself to deep breathe immediately. With practice, this often sends you back to sleep without too much disturbance.

Hot weather

A heatwave can overwork the heart by up to two-thirds, because as the body tries to adapt to the temperature, the heart has to work harder to pump blood to the body surface through the skin. In very high temperatures the body also sweats to lose heat, thereby losing salt and water, leading to body fluids, especially the blood, becoming more concentrated, stickier and more likely to clot. Add in the natural occurrence of age, where the body is less able to adapt to conditions of hot and cold, with the added consequence of coronary heart disease (CHD), and you can see the increasing strain put on your heart.

Here are some helpful suggestions:

- In hot weather wear lightweight, light-coloured cotton clothes because pale colours reflect the sun's radiation better than dark ones.
- Drink plenty of fluids, particularly water. Keep a jug in the fridge and top up your glass at least every hour.
- Wear a hat or cap in the sun and cover the sensitive areas of your body. The night before you go out for a day, roll up some damp flannels and pop them in the freezer. Take them with you in a plastic bag. When you start to feel hot, unwrap them and place them over your face, neck or wrists.
- If you like to sunbathe, do not go out in the hottest part of the day. Early morning or late afternoon are best, but always make sure that any scar tissue from an operation is covered up (it can be very sensitive to heat). Wait 20 minutes for suncream to be absorbed and stay in direct sunlight for no longer than one hour at a time.
- If you feel hot, place your wrists under cool water, as running water applied directly to 'pulse points' draws the heat out of your blood even if the water isn't particularly cold itself.

3

Coping with emotions

Just look at what you have been through. Hasn't it had its traumatic moments? Have you been constantly trying to put on a brave face and pretend everything is OK? If you have, what good has it done you? The following processes will definitely help the 'brave face brigade', but even those of you who allow yourselves to show emotion will find the techniques useful. Later on in this book we'll explore more in-depth ways of analysing your feelings and behaviour patterns so as to enhance your recovery, but for now, why not give these suggestions a go – they certainly won't harm you.

Loss

Are you surprised that I include a section on loss in this book? Some of you may be, but I guess most of you will say, 'No, that's just how I feel – empty, lost, unsure, fearful of upsetting others, or being judged by others as weak, not being able to stop once I start crying, and seeing myself as weak for doing so.'

We all experience minor or devastating emotion with loss – in this case, the loss of what we were before a heart condition changed our lives. But if the natural outpouring is continually suppressed, illness is often the result. Those of you who have experienced a loss of a close loved one, but who believed they needed to be strong to support others, may immediately identify with this. Loss can be perceived in three ways:

Actual	e.g. someone or something we knew or loved (loss of limb, loss of mobility)
Perceived	e.g. inability to look after myself or my family
Feared	e.g. never be able to be normal again (fear that heart attack may return or condition worsen)

While everyone accepts your feelings about an 'actual' loss, the other two tend to generate responses like 'Don't worry, just forget about it'. Yet illnesses such as a heart condition can generate great feelings of loss which, if suppressed, will hinder the recovery process.

Emotional upheaval is a natural side effect of any treatment. Expectations that you should be able to cope, or fears that you will not be able to do so, will ebb and flow as the days, weeks and months fly by. If this is not the case for you, I would be concerned, because the likelihood is you would be suppressing your fears instead of dealing with them. As already discussed, your recovery will be affected if you constantly bottle things up (known in the 'stress trade' as 'avoidance practice'), so here are some ways to let those feelings out, safely.

Crying

Crying is a natural human process, the same for men and women, seen as normal in childhood but frequently perceived as weak in adulthood. Yet scientific facts show things differently. When we cry, a chemical called enkaphalin (or ankaphalin), the body's natural sedative, is released, ultimately calming us. If we keep trying to hold back tears we get pain behind the eyes, a choking feeling in the throat, and other feelings such as stomach rumbles, rashes, shakes and feelings of tension or agitation. Your recovery needs you to release those emotions. Whenever you feel like crying, say to yourself, 'I have a right to cry, and if I want to, I'm going to.'

How does it work? Physiologically, the body is releasing unhealthy emotions before they get to the pressured stage. I use this all the time and I cry very rarely, not because I think it is weak, but because I let myself whenever I need too. Remember such a belief statement also releases serotonin, the mind's 'happy' chemical.

For those of you who fear that seeing you cry may upset others, there are two things you can do. First, whenever you feel emotional, go to the loo, sit there, and give yourself permission to cry; second, 'set the scene' by saying to others, 'When I feel bad, I realize I need to let the emotion out, so if I start crying, don't worry, just let me be. I feel better afterwards.' This gives permission to express emotions to others as well as to ourselves.

Remember to use 'the right to cry' as often as you feel the need. With time, you will cry less and feel so much better, allowing your immune system to work on the physical instead of emotional needs of your body. Everyone I know who has tried this has come back and said, 'I feel so much better' and 'I can't believe it, I've cried less'.

Writing a letter

Sometimes people feel unable to describe their loss verbally. In this case, they can write a letter to themselves, expressing their fears and anxieties. Unlike crying, this need only be done once, and this letter is not intended for you to show to others, although where couples have both written down their feelings and allowed the other to read them, they have achieved greater understanding of each other's feelings. While you may find it difficult, completing such a letter can bring a tremendous release of emotion.

You need a quiet space – no interruptions, no television, no radio, phone off the hook, and definitely a box of tissues. Start with a heading such as 'What I have lost' or 'Having a heart condition, what it means to me' and then begin to write how you feel right now, not the story of what happened, until you can write no more.

How much you write is irrelevant; it can be one paragraph or many pages. Nearly everyone reflects on the difficulty of completing such a process, but when they do, they also express a sense of relief. When completed, read it only once, seal it in an envelope, and put it away.

'Binning'

You can use a similar process whenever emotional difficulties such as anger, anxiety, guilt, frustration, irritability or depression lead to that 'wound-up feeling'. I call this 'binning', a stress-reducing technique.

Janice

Janice spoke of great distress because of her illness. 'I just can't stand not being able to do what I normally do. I feel so useless, pathetic, stupid and angry with everybody around me.' Whenever she felt like this, Janice was asked to write down exactly what she was thinking, using any words she wanted. Once she had written it, she had to finish with a realistic positive sentence we had worked on together, such as, 'OK, I'm frustrated, that's normal, but every day I'm getting stronger. Great, the rubbish is out; now let's replace it with something good for me.'

Reading it only once she folded it and tore it into tiny pieces, throwing it into the bin. She said, 'At first I couldn't understand why it was working, I just felt less agitated, and then I found myself repeating that last sentence over and over again and I do now feel stronger.'

Writing down feelings and tearing them up allows the mind to release persistent, negative thoughts. This process is not about taking the emotion away so that it never bothers you again. This is not possible – we are human! But it is about taking away the intensity that inhibits your well-being. I use this process whenever I feel something in my life is unfair, or I'm particularly upset or angry. It's great, it belongs to me, I share with it with no one, and I love that tearing-up bit!

Accepting yourself

Learn to accept yourself as you are, as you have been, and as you can be. Known as 'self-acceptability', this is a powerful tool because it means that we are not continuously striving to be 'perfect', with a corresponding fear of failing.

Self-acceptance is a kind of 'umbrella' or protective shield against outside influences or the bombardment of the internal 'self-doubt hammer'. It also means accepting responsibility for stress in our lives because we can take the trauma out of a crisis by 'owning' our part in it.

At this time you are undoubtedly already aware of your clinical needs and any personal limitations. Learning to accept your situation, and the limitations imposed by recovery, enables you to review the possible changes you can make to ensure on-going preventative care. As your strength develops, your range of possibilities will broaden, but only if you accept who you are at this time.

How to accept yourself

1 *Acknowledge* your difficulty at this time, e.g. being unable to do your garden.
2 *Allow* and *Accept* the emotions that ensue, e.g. it's all right to feel annoyed, upset and frustrated – and let these feelings out.
3 *Use* the constructive tools in this book to challenge and diminish the effects of any unrealistic beliefs.

Accepting yourself also ties in with beliefs about how a job should be done. If you are someone who believes that 'It's got to be perfect or it's not good enough', you will constantly question the outcome and, I suspect, hammer away at yourself if you feel it isn't good enough, creating intense pressure and unrealistic expectations.

Challenging such thoughts will enhance your recovery. For example, say to yourself, 'I want to do this well, and I'm going to take time to do so, but as long as I know I've given it my best shot, that's all that matters.'

Living alone

Do you live alone? Some people are content with their own company, but others feel lonely. Living alone during an illness can be depressing and scary, especially if you are experiencing uncomfortable side effects of any medication. If this is the case, do tell your coronary care nurse or doctor, who can sort out medication issues and who should have access to voluntary organizations and support groups. If not, you can contact the BHF (see Useful addresses) for local coronary support groups, or your local council for contact details of relevant organizations. Some of these organizations have volunteers who will sit with you for short periods while you are recovering. When you feel better, getting out and socializing is the greatest lifter of moods. Perhaps you like to help others and, if so, you could consider joining a voluntary group yourself when you feel strong enough. The skills and knowledge you have gained, especially perhaps during your illness, will be of benefit to others.

Even if you don't feel alone, you can still feel isolated because you believe that others, who have not shared your experience, do not understand how you feel. In this case, joining a coronary support group gives you the chance to meet those with similar experiences of coronary heart disease. You can also take a family member with you (very beneficial to them) and learn more about different aspects of coronary heart disease through talks given by medical practitioners, nurses, other people with heart disease, and others. There may also be social and fund-raising events such as quiz nights, as well as coronary rehabilitation courses and walking programmes. For example, the last course I presented involved a review called 'Heart Disease from a Partner's Perspective'. Just remember the pace and symptoms of the healing process tend not to be the same for everyone, therefore listening to others' experiences and ways they cope is best viewed as an opportunity to reflect on your situation and coping mechanisms, not an absolute. The last thing you want is to emerge from such a talk saying, 'I must now feel or do as they do.'

Relationships

One of the most difficult problems for people still reeling from the shock of their diagnosis or treatment is how to share feelings without worrying others or being perceived as odd, inadequate, weak, unattractive and even replaceable.

If you find it easy to communicate how you feel, that's great. Use the following as a constructive reminder of the skills you already have.

If, however, you identify with any of the following, practising ways to communicate better will really help your recovery:

- Are you concerned because you tend to over-elaborate, wanting to go into too much detail, while listeners may appear bored or disinterested?
- Conversely, do you tend to be too short and sharp in your descriptions, so that others appear confused and may question what you mean?
- Or do you just find it difficult to find the words to express yourself?

How to change

Accept that negative feelings and thoughts are normal, no matter how extreme they seem, but suppressing them effectively slows down the healing process. This is not to suggest you 'have to' share such thoughts and feelings with others. Let them out, yes, use the 'binning' technique mentioned previously, but if you're worried about anyone reading it, write the feelings down in private and then burn them or throw them away, or even lock yourself into the loo to write, and then flush your notes down the toilet.

Try sharing your feelings by first 'setting the scene'. Be honest with family and friends: 'Look, at the moment my mind keeps racing and I feel very emotional, but it helps me to say what I'm thinking and feeling. Don't worry if I get upset – I just need to let it out.'

Carers worry more if you say nothing, as their imagination may lead them to think the worst, and perhaps constantly question how you are. This is very frustrating if you can't, or don't want to, explain how you feel.

The 'I' exercise

If you have difficulty finding words to express yourself, try this exercise:

Write down one word that describes the way you feel physically at the moment, e.g. 'tired'; one word that describes how you feel emotionally at the moment, e.g. 'miserable'; one word to describe the feelings that keep coming into your mind, e.g. 'unfair'; and one word that describes your behaviour, e.g. 'avoiding'. Now put all these words together, i.e. tired, miserable, unfair and avoiding.

Now put them into a sentence that begins with the word 'I': 'I am tired, miserable and avoiding people because it's so unfair I've got this – why me?'

As you can see, I began the sentence with 'I', which is an invaluable assertive and communicative tool to use when you want to tell others how you feel. Try explaining your thoughts by using 'I' at the beginning of as many sentences as you can. It creates a tendency to listen on the part of the receiver and a feeling of being in control at your end. For example, look at the sentences below. One is demanding or fault-finding, while the other expresses an opinion. Which one would you prefer to hear and which would you be more likely to positively respond to?

- 'You're not listening to me' as opposed to 'I feel as if no one is listening to me properly'.
- 'None of you understands how this feels' as opposed to 'I just feel so tired, I want to sleep all the time'.

You and others

Partners can sometimes take each other for granted through familiarity and perhaps complacency, but at times of intense uncertainty and fear, this natural state of affairs needs to be reviewed.

Reflect for a moment. Do you tend to talk to each other while doing other things, or do you sit down and talk? The latter is what you need to do now.

Happily, most people do feel supported by their family – in fact, 97 per cent of those in my coronary survey reported that their relationship was strengthened. Those of you who find being at home has highlighted some problems would benefit from reviewing the following communication skills:

- Go back to using the basic form of communication, touch. Allow and seek out comfort from cuddles and hugs.
- Make eye contact with your partner before you start talking.
- Allow sufficient time to talk. Stop what you are doing and sit down together.
- Talk through your problems. Listen to each other without interrupting.
- Whenever you feel agitated take a deep breath before you respond to a comment from your partner or a family member. It will give you time to think about your response and help you to feel less tense.
- The more agitated and loud your response is, the more the discussion is likely to develop into an argument. Try to keep your tone as calm and controlled as you can. Remember, breathing properly definitely helps.
- Where older children and teenagers are concerned, you need to accept that your ideas and way of living are not necessarily what they wish to follow. Have your say, express your views, and then accept that they, just like you, need to live their own lives.
- Plan a budget together that covers all your expenses, particularly if you may be unable to return to work. Include working children in this discussion. Stress often results when only one person is dealing with a situation, especially if he or she is trying to cover up money problems.
- If you are unable to reach a solution together, seek professional guidance, either from associations such as Relate or counsellors who work with couples.
- Going out may seem the last thing you want to do while recovering, but it is a great relationship 'bonder'. Choose places to go that you both like, will not be overcrowded or involve extensive walking (initially), and seek to go out once a week. Start with a short one- or two-hour jaunt and, as you feel stronger, lengthen the time.
- Many, if not most, of you reading this book are parents, and some will be grandparents. Share your knowledge of your newly learnt skills to help your children, and grandchildren, to live healthier lives.

For carers

Caring for a family member who is or has been ill can be extremely stressful as it is often a prolonged process, made worse if you are not living with the person who has coronary heart disease. Most carers, certainly initially, tend to over-compensate for the needs of the person recovering, without focusing on their own needs. We have already seen how important it is for those recovering from coronary heart disease to prioritize their own needs in order to restore their energies; it is exactly the same for you, the carer. There are many aspects of the sick person's recovery period upon which it would benefit you to reflect, such as the following:

- You need to accept that they have been, and in some cases still are, ill. Also accept that you cannot take their pain away but you can support them to help themselves, so that they not only recover from their present illness, but also undertake long-term preventative health measures.
- Recognize your limitations and ensure you have time for yourself to recharge your own batteries. Allow others to support you (and your partner), even if it is only a few hours' break. If you do not have a friend or family member to help, there are many organizations that provide volunteers either to sit with your partner or to complete a chore for you.
- Lessen any worries or fears by talking to family or friends. Try out yourself all the suggestions I have detailed in this book – they work for you, too.
- Talk to the person who is recovering, and don't hide your feelings – he or she may share your fears and also need to talk.
- If the person recovering appears unwell, talk to your doctor no matter how trivial it may seem. Sometimes it is your fear that is generating concern, not the actual recovery of the person.
- One of the greatest fears for carers is, 'Is my recovering partner or family member doing too much?' Join a coronary exercise class together. It allays fears and gets *you* fit into the bargain!
- Above all, be positive and happy that the person has returned home. Remember, he or she would not have been sent home unless the doctor considered he/she were fit enough to do so.
- Once the early stages of recovery are over, work together on any pursuit or project, e.g. go for a walk or join an adult education class together, or undertake joint activities such as redecorating – especially important if your partner was the type to do everything

himself or herself before the illness.

- One of the most natural responses to a person's voiced fears is to immediately give a positive answer. While this can indeed be helpful, in my experience it is more helpful *not* to. However, I do not mean keep quiet and say nothing! Instead, get the other person to provide the answer himself. For example, David might say to his partner, Claire, 'This pain in my chest really catches me.' Instead of Claire replying, 'Oh, that's normal, it's OK,' or, 'You'd better go straight to the doctor,' she could try saying, 'What did they tell you at the hospital to do about such pain?' David may reply, 'Oh, that I should expect it. It's not a heart attack, it's a muscular spasm around the scar tissue.' See the difference. By saying it himself, he hears it and believes it, whereas sometimes when others provide the answer, we may just think they are either being dismissive or trying to be nice.

4

Dealing with stress in recovery

Resuming normal life is naturally very important, but often this means the need to change, sometimes drastically, behaviours that may have fuelled your susceptibility towards developing a heart condition. This involves taking a close look at stress – not just in general, but how it may have affected you personally.

Obviously I sincerely hope this book will prove an invaluable recovery tool for you, but also it can help you to create your own more *personalized* recovery book.

So at this stage I'd suggest you get yourself a small notebook and write down any of the coping skills that particularly relate to you, as well as any tips from others, so as to make your own 'Coaching Myself to Health Book'.

How does stress affect the immune system and heart?

Our immune systems protect our metabolism against attacks from bacteria, viruses and cancer cells, but their effectiveness can be inhibited by certain stimuli. One of the main stimuli is persistent, intense stress, or 'burn-out', a state of physical, emotional and mental exhaustion that results from long-term involvement in work/life situations that are relentless, resulting in the development of both physical and psychological illness.

Has this happened to you in the past? Are you experiencing it now? Do you fear it for the future? Do you believe stress has affected your heart condition? If so, read on and see why evidence suggests it might have done.

What is stress?

The stress response is an inherent part of us, developed to release chemicals known as noradrenaline (in control, ready to fight) and adrenaline (out of control, fleeing) – energy resources to either fight our attacker or flee to safety. Today, although we still have this stress response, and indeed face increased numbers and different types of threats and challenges, we are often unable to fully release the stress created within our bodies. Over a period of time, this progressive stress eventually creates intense suppression, so fuelling a predisposition towards ill health.

Many people find it difficult to comprehend how stress is felt. To help, I use the following imagery:

Imagine there is a spring inside you, naturally bouncing away when you feel good, tightening up a bit when you need to focus, but releasing when the task is completed (i.e. *normal pressure)*.

Now imagine that spring getting more and more wound up as you feel more and more pressurized, until it just seems to explode, either with outbursts of anger/tears, feeling exhausted, avoidance or illness (i.e. *unmanageable pressure*).

Now look at Figure 1. Which one of the diagrams was you before your diagnosis, during your illness and after medical intervention?

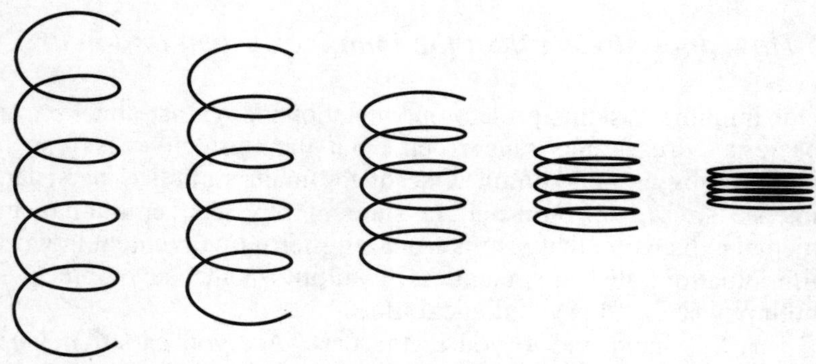

Figure 1 Various coiled springs demonstrating degrees of stress

The first spring is normal, bouncing up and down as we need it every day; the second spring is tighter, showing what happens internally when we are focused or active; the third spring relates to unmanageable pressure, tension and discomfort; the fourth spring relates to great distress, and is frequently chosen by those who have illnesses or disease; the fifth spring relates to overload in all aspects of an individual's life, leading to burn-out. This 'wind-up' process, while felt physically, is often stimulated by something we think, see, feel, hear, taste or smell. It is a reactive process that is different for each individual – what 'winds up' one person won't necessarily do the same to another.

How can stress specifically affect your recovery?

First, it can affect your ability to take on board medical advice because stress restricts our attention to events around us. Even when information is clearly given, mental, physical, behavioural and emotional stressors can inhibit our ability to decipher, retain and act upon it.

Second, after surgery, your level of stress could affect the healing process, because it increases production of the stress hormones noradrenaline and cortisol, which can trigger inflammation and slow the wound-healing process by up to 40 per cent.

Third, while it is natural and normal to have mood swings after illness, there can be an enormous pendulum swing from high elation through to tears and even depression, leading to fear of losing control and making your heart condition worse. In essence, the complexity of our make-up means that any physical symptoms of illness or distress are interlinked with the way we think, the way we behave and the emotional consequences of inactive or active practice.

Fourth, the effects of work, environmental, relationship, health and social stresses will impinge and affect all aspects of our lives. For example, exposure to stress for at least half our working life means we are 25 per cent more likely to have a heart attack, and 50 per cent more likely to suffer a stroke. Research shows that 2 per cent of men in their forties and fifties suffer abnormal heart rhythms caused by stress, exhaustion or even consuming too much caffeine.

Therefore finding ways of recognizing symptoms and dealing with stress is an essential element of your recovery process. Even if your levels of stress are manageable, you would benefit from reviewing the coping strategies I detail in this book.

Stopping pressure turning into stress

Stress is not something that occurs just because you have become ill; it is constant in our lives, a normal process, and only needs dealing with when it is identified as unmanageable. So first we need to ascertain how stress affects you personally:

Look at the material in Table 4.1 and, using different-coloured pens, make a note of the physical, emotional, behavioural and mental outcomes or triggers of stress that:

- Have affected you in the past.
- You believe fuelled the development of your heart condition.
- Affect you at this time.
- Are most severe at this time.

You can add any others you can think of. Interesting, isn't it! These are all normal reactions that we all have, yet when we review them in this way we can see how stress varies in the form it takes.

Adam

Even before learning about his illness, Adam was prone to physical symptoms such as headaches, neck aches, palpitations, excessive sweating, clenched jaw and restlessness – he was unable to keep still. He tended to blame others or himself, became easily distracted, worried all the time in case he made a mistake and had persistent negative thoughts, becoming easily agitated, tense, alienated from his colleagues and unhappy with his job. Ultimately he became aggressive, over-ate, had disturbed sleep and didn't have time to relax. Small wonder that he often ended up feeling depressed and worn out.

Adam believed that tension, frustration (often self-created) and stress at work had fuelled his heart condition because he was always working late trying to get things done – not just his own work, but others' work too.

When we reviewed the triggers that were still affecting him, he pinpointed feelings of continued impatience with himself and his own family. He would become tense and angry and start shouting, which would in turn make his chest hurt, at which point he blamed himself! Indeed, Adam's outbursts began the whole distressing spiral all over again, leading to further distress and

Table 4.1 The various forms that stress can take

Physical	*Mental*	*Emotional*	*Behavioural*
Unable to keep still	Blaming of self or others	Agitated, sullen	Aggressive
Headaches	Indecision	Irritability	Being unsocial
Indigestion	Memory failing	More gloomy, depressed	Restlessness
Breathlessness	Easily distracted	Drained, no enthusiasm	Loss of appetite or over-eating
Palpitations	Loss of concentration	Feeling tense	Poor time-keeping
Nausea	Bad dreams	Cynical, feeling guilty	Increase or decrease in sexual desire
Tiredness	Worrying	Alienated	Bad driving
Vague aches or pains	Muddled thinking	Feeling nervous, apprehensive	Disturbed sleep
Skin irritation or eczema	Making mistakes	Anxious	Drinking more
Excessive sweating	Less intuitive	Feeling of pointlessness	Taking work home
Clenched fist or jaw	Less sensitive	Loss of confidence	Too busy to relax, impatient
Diarrhoea	Persistent negative thoughts	Less satisfaction in life	Not looking after oneself
Cold hands and feet	Demotivated	Totally distracted, easily forget things	Accident prone, scream and shout excessively
Neck aches	Over-sensitivity, under-valuing oneself	Reduced self-esteem, job dissatisfaction	Lying, unable to unwind
Feeling dizzy	Finding fault with others	Crying easily	Low productivity
Butterfly stomach or dry mouth	Expecting things to be done	Get easily frustrated, angry	Increased problems at home

Table 4.2 Sources of stress and their ratings

Situation	*Level of stress (graded 1 to 10)*	*Persistent thoughts*	*Image*
Is it personal, the way you think, feel about yourself or your condition?	10+	'You're useless, and everyone thinks so too'	Very tight spring
To do with work?	9	'They should be doing their own work and then I wouldn't get so wound up'	
Family?	7	'They expect so much of me, I can see it in their eyes'	
Friends?	6	'I have to keep up appearances even when I'm shattered'	
The environment where you live	4	'It's great here, no one around to bother me or ask me to do anything'	
Money worries	8	'I have to work or we can't keep going, it costs so much to live'	
Lack of confidence	6	'I don't let them see I'm afraid; I keep up the front'	
Driving	7	'How stupid you are: learn to drive or get off the road'	
Any fears (heights, etc.)	4	'I'm only afraid of not getting things done, nothing else scares me'	

eventually complete exhaustion, when he would have to go to bed.

Back to you, can you see your connectors? Write them down as Adam did.

Now you need to identify the source of stress, i.e. in what circumstances, and when, how and where it occurs and, having written down these sources:

- Grade the severity of stress for each one at this time from one to ten, ten being the worst.
- Think about any persistent thoughts that tend to be around during times of stress.
- Think of an image that for you describes what being stressed feels like. If you can, name it and draw it.

Table 4.2, opposite, gives an example of a chart you could use, and Adam's responses.

Once you are aware of what causes a situation to become stressful you can learn to reduce its harmful impact on your health.

Dealing with stressors

Professor Stephen Palmer devised the following checklist as a tool to help people identify already learnt coping skills, calling them *stability zones* and *rituals/routines*.

Stability zones

These are areas where an individual may be able to relax, feel safe and be able to forget about worries, for example:

- Home with or without the family.
- Holiday home/caravan.
- Park.
- Special place at home.
- Beach.
- Favourite pub, restaurant, café, chair, country walk, old car, old clothes.

Rituals/routines

These are enjoyable regular or irregular habits or routines that individuals may have in their tool bag of coping mechanisms. However, these rituals are not to the point of obsession. Some examples are:

- Walking the dog.
- Morning cup of tea.
- Hobbies, i.e. gardening.
- Weekend breaks.
- Eating out once a week.
- Sunday outings.
- Holidays.
- Watching old films.
- Talking with/meeting old friends.

I have often used such checklists to establish ways for people to reduce stress in their lives. For example, members of my coronary group identified the following stability zones and rituals/routines where they are able to relax, feel safe and try to forget their worries:

- 'I'm most relaxed when I am in my conservatory, I just love looking out at my garden. I soak up the view, and I love the sounds of the birds and the rain. I often fall asleep in there, which is good because I don't sleep well.'
- 'I love my bed. I feel safe there and can read to my heart's content.'
- 'I love walking, being out in the fresh air. Even when I'm not feeling well, going outside and breathing in that air makes me feel better.'
- 'The most relaxing place for me is in my home. Also, having a cup of tea and telling my partner how I'm feeling. She's a very good listener.'
- 'I love my old car, cleaning it, listening to the sound of the engine and occasionally driving it.'

Write down in your 'Coaching Myself to Health Book' your own stability zones and rituals/routines and ensure you use them. They will provide invaluable comfort, relaxation and reassurance on your route to recovery.

5

Diaphragmatic breathing

Of all the techniques I show people, no matter what their age or difficulties, this is the one that everyone likes the best. It is instantaneous, can be practised anywhere at any time, costs nothing, gives immediate release from tension, and creates a feeling of being in control.

Benefits of diaphragmatic breathing

Breathing is the first and last thing we do in our lives, an automatic process, controlled – like all our other internal functions – by the autonomic nervous system. It is a natural process that cannot be stopped by holding the breath, but can be enhanced through diaphragmatic breathing, which helps create a deeper breath and induce a calmer state. Breathing also stimulates and assists circulation by acting as a vacuum, sucking up blood from the feet and legs back to the heart.

Diaphragmatic breathing:

- Uses the lungs efficiently.
- Reduces the workload for the heart and its need for increased oxygen. Releases tension and stress.
- Promotes stamina.
- Encourages effective sleep patterns.
- Increases the capacity of the muscles to work harder and longer.
- Relaxes the body, and encourages positive thoughts and belief in your ability to deal with your condition.

Diaphragmatic breathing is developed through the full use of chest muscles pulling the ribs up and down, enabling a better intake of fresh oxygen, which is passed through the lungs and pumped by the heart to organs and working muscles, and forces carbon dioxide, the waste product of respiration, out of the lungs.

Emotional and physical aspects of shallow breathing

Although our lungs fill our breast cavity and are designed to be fully used, often we shallow breathe, which is more likely to encourage tension, anxiety, tightness in the chest, panicky feelings and fatigue. Breathlessness can also be caused by physical exertion, high altitudes, anaemia, an overactive thyroid gland, asthma or emphysema.

Breathing difficulties may be related to your medical condition, to other illnesses, or to a tendency to become anxious.

It is essential to understand that there is a difference between shallow breathing induced by illness, and shallow breathing brought on by emotional stress. Don't try and self-diagnose. Consult your GP if you are worried about your breathing.

The following are recognised consequences of shallow breathing:

- Breathing rapidly and often when anxious.
- Sighing frequently when feeling depressed.
- Anxious individuals tend to talk at the peak of inhalation, while depressed individuals tend to talk at the end of exhalation.
- When feeling angry or fearful, breathing becomes irregular and mainly shallow.

Persistent shallow breathing stops the heart from receiving its most vital fuel, oxygen, and this leads to fatigue, tension headaches, a rapid heartbeat (palpitations), sweating, dizziness or fainting. The problem may be worsened by soreness and pain from a surgery scar, which can in itself cause shallow breathing. Taking cold air in through the mouth causes a sensation of tightness in the chest, leading to even shallower breaths. This in turn leads to a tendency to over-breathe, caused by the fear of not getting enough oxygen.

Shallow breathing and anxiety

These are often linked and shallow breathing can sometimes lead to panic attacks. Perhaps you yourself have experienced anxiety where the heart races, or panic attacks where you felt as if you were unable to breathe.

As human beings we are stimulated by our six senses: the way we think, hear, see, feel, taste and smell. These stimulants can trigger a reaction to 'catch' our breath with either shock or fear, leading to a surge of adrenaline from the hypothalamus, which races to the heart and makes the heart beat faster. The mind quickly picks up this physical reaction and fearful thoughts begin to surface, leading to even shallower breaths, fuelling further adrenaline surges and so on until the person believes he or she cannot breathe (a full-blown panic attack).

> ***Michael***
> Michael was concerned because he needed to have an ECG. All day long he was thinking about this and was occasionally aware that his heart was racing. When he got to the hospital and his heart started to beat very loudly, he caught his breath with concern and thought, 'I'm having a heart attack.' He began to panic, his heart raced faster, he caught his breath again, felt he couldn't breathe, and collapsed on the floor.

One woman told me how she was diagnosed at 40 with low blood pressure, and then hospitalized. She experienced many of the unpleasant symptoms described above, until she began to practise my relaxation and deep breathing exercises. Feeling much better, she began a programme of yoga, exercise and swimming and, within a year, her blood pressure had reached normal levels and has remained so ever since.

Contraindications to diaphragmatic breathing

There are situations where diaphragmatic breathing may be difficult. For example, if you suffer from asthma, anxiety attacks, have a smoker's cough or are recovering from by-pass surgery (where the scar tissue and breast bone will initially be sore), deep breathing can be difficult, not because you can't do it, but because you fear doing it.

Although none of the above have caused problems for those who work with me, if you are aware of any of these difficulties, ensure that you talk to someone experienced in teaching diaphragmatic breathing who can help you to create a breathing regime to suit your needs.

Check your natural breathing rhythm

Ensure you are seated comfortably with your feet grounded. Your back should be pushed firmly into the back of the chair, with your arms resting on your lap or the arms of the chair.

Place one hand above your breast or on your chest and one hand on your diaphragm (just under your ribcage).

Breathe normally. Which hand moves, the top or bottom one? If the top hand moved, you are more prone to shallow breathing, and if the bottom hand moved you are more prone to deep breathing. Sometimes people feel that both moved; if this happens, close your eyes and try again.

You should now have an idea of your natural breathing rhythm.

Deep breathing

Try the following:

Place your hand on your diaphragm or stomach, take a deep breath in through your nose, feeling the area under your hand fill up just like a balloon; immediately it feels full, breathe out hard and long through your mouth. Repeat this twice more.

Try it again but this time close your eyes – it helps to feel the sensation better.

How do you feel now? Most people say they now feel calmer and more relaxed; occasionally, they say that they found it difficult. Did you feel any sensation of dizziness? Don't worry if you did: this is often related to not exhaling deeply enough before you take the next breath. Just ensure you inhale and exhale fully and slowly with the exhaled breath being longer.

Occasionally people find it difficult to get the in and out rhythm right, in which case you can try a counting rhythm which ensures that the out breath is longer than the in: e.g. Place your hand on your diaphragm or stomach, and take a breath in, two, three, four, and out, two, three, four, five; and in, two, three, four, and out, two, three, four, five.

Whether you count or not, it is essential that you feel a natural rhythm from the in to the out breath.

Imagery and deep breathing

Using imagery can also help you to develop your ability to deep breathe. Try the following exercise: Imagine the in breath is like filling up a balloon and the out breath is like letting the air go from that balloon – it is more explosive.

Once you've learnt how to do it, deep calming breathing needs to become an everyday occurrence, not just when you feel anxious, in pain or fearful, but also to feel good and relaxed. I frequently take deep breaths when I am working on my computer, and at the moment I've just taken some extra ones!

Making it an everyday skill

1 Put the letter B (for breathe) on the handset of your phone (at home, at work and on a mobile) and every time the phone rings do not answer it until you have taken one deep breath. People I know who have stressful jobs say this technique is their favourite one, because they recognize the difference it makes to their voice when they answer the phone, and they feel calmer and more in control. Even if the caller is irritating them, they just put their hand over the mouthpiece and deep breathe while the other person is speaking. Try it.
2 Take several deep breaths whenever a situation or thought creates an awareness of feeling either tense or anxious.
3 Use a health-enhancing thought as you breathe in and out; for example, as you breathe in, think, 'Fresh oxygen in.' As you breathe out, think, 'Wasted energy out.'

Situations where deep breathing can help

Now let's explore specific situations where deep breathing, either on its own or with other coping strategies, can assist your recovery. All of these examples have been taken from the experiences of coronary rehabilitation participants.

Getting out of bed

When you are at the initial stage of recovery it can feel scary and getting out of bed will probably pull on your chest if you have undergone surgery. If you have been lying down for some time, it can also create a dizzy sensation as you get up. All this is perfectly normal. Breathing will help, but initially you may, because of soreness on the chest, need to practise it without the deep breathing processes I have already described.

When you first wake up become acclimatized to your surroundings and then take two deep breaths, as deep as is comfortable for you. If you have difficulty getting out of bed or feel anxious about doing so, try this:

- Ensure your covers are light and not tucked in.
- Take a breath in through your nose, as deeply as you comfortably can, while at the same time moving your knees towards you until they are bent, and breathe out as you place your feet firmly on the mattress.
- Wait a moment.
- When you are ready, take another breath in, and as you breathe out roll over on to your side, one whole movement, shoulders, hips and knees all at the same time. (If you suffer from arthritic pain that makes movement difficult, gently rock the body to and fro until you have the momentum to roll over. If carers are assisting you, they need to gently place their hands on your shoulder and knee and rock with you until they can generate with a gentle pull your movement on to your side.)
- Wait a moment.
- When you are ready, take another breath and, as you breathe out, allow your legs to swing or drop down over the side of your bed.
- Wait a moment.
- When you are ready, take another breath and slowly push up to a sitting position (use your elbow and then your hand for support).
- Allow the body to settle, just sit there for a moment and, when you are ready, take four deep breaths in and out before you get up. (Remember, any dizziness you experience means you have either been lying still for too long or you have taken too much fresh oxygen in and not let the stale oxygen out.) Wait until any dizziness subsides before you rise.

If you haven't had any treatment yet, practise this now before you go into hospital as practice is the key to managing discomfort or pain.

Driving

Today, driving seems to provoke a great deal more anxiety than in the past because of our fast pace of living, resulting in loss of concentration, agitation, tension and sometimes anger. Deep breathing linked to a simple shoulder exercise is an effective way to deal with such emotions, even if you are just the passenger. In fact, many rehab patients find being a passenger is far worse than driving! Try this:

- Take several deep breaths before you get into the car. If recovering from an operation when your body is sore, sit down with your legs outside the car and then take a breath in at the same time as you breathe out, swing your legs and turn your upper body into the car.
- Before you put your seat belt on, take one deep breath, raising your shoulders towards your ears, circle them back and down as you breathe out, resting your back securely against your seat. If you have scar soreness, bring a little cushion with you to place under the seat beat.
- Any time you feel tense in the car and appear to be sitting forwards, repeat the breathing and the shoulder circling action.
- If you are driving, ensure you are comfortable and repeat the processes as above.

Discomfort or pain after surgery

Be realistic: it will feel uncomfortable, even hurt at times, when you breathe; this is related to scar tissue, bruising around the operated area, and natural anxiety. Gradually increase the depth of the breath until a peak of comfort is reached before it hurts and then immediately expel the air. Eventually the skin will stretch and the soreness will ease.

Getting dressed

Getting dressed in the mornings can be difficult. Do not hold your breath. Take a breath in as you put on a piece of clothing, and breathe out as you pull it down.

Remember this catchphrase:

Hold your breath, pain increases
Breathe through pain and it eases

If, however, you have any concern related to continuing pain or discomfort, go and see your GP.

Posture and breathing

Posture promotes balance, and demonstrates confidence, vitality and a sense of well-being. Therefore the way you sit or stand can affect your recovery. When recovering from an injury or operation there is a natural tendency to compensate for any discomfort by using another part of the body to take the weight, using a stick to walk (which means people tend to lean to one side) or allowing the body to hunch up, usually with shoulders leaning forwards. Such postural changes can become fixed if they are incessantly used. What can you do about it?

Imagine you have a strong pin right through your middle, coming out of the head (like a puppet). Its strength enables every other part of the body to move easily. Whenever you recognize your body is not straight, take a deep breath and put it back in alignment. With practice, the healing process will be enhanced as your weight is evenly distributed and therefore the support is greater.

Getting up out of a chair

If you are on your own

Choose a chair that is firm, and with firm cushions and armrests. Place your feet slightly apart and stand as tall as you can. Place your hands on the armrests as you slowly sit down. When you want to get up, wiggle your bottom towards the edge of the chair. Place your hands firmly on the armrests, take a breath in, and as you breathe out push up with your hands. Wait a moment, take a couple of deep breaths, and then walk.

Information for carers

Stand in front of the person sitting down and place one foot between their feet, with the other back and to one side. Place your hands firmly under the person's elbows and get them to place theirs under yours. Take a deep breath and, as you breathe out, lower your arms and bend at the knees. Encourage the person sitting down to wiggle their bottom towards the edge of the chair; then, once there, gently rock forwards and backwards (your feet, remember, are one in front of the other). Both of you in unison then take a deep breath, and as the sitter breathes out, they rise up, with the carer gently stepping back until their feet are side by side. In effect, you are taking the sitter's weight, which is why you need to bend at the knees (reduces lower back strain).

Muscular/back pain and breathing

This is something that many of us experience, particularly when we get older, as our postural habits mean we sit badly. For example, as I am typing this book, I often become aware of a pain in my neck. I know this means I am sitting badly. As soon as this happens, I stop what I am doing, uncurl my feet (very common, but inhibits circulation), sit on the edge of the seat, and slowly wiggle my bottom towards the back of the chair. When my bottom touches the back, I slowly allow the rest of my body to uncurl. Immediately my posture is improved and my neck ache is reduced. I then take four deep breaths and I can begin typing again. Try it, preferably in a firm chair.

Whatever you do, remember you're normal and, just like me, will return to your seemingly comfortable but actually bad habitual posture. But whenever you become aware of your posture being wrong, change it.

Pain on walking

This can be a problem for some, particularly if you have angina or leg pain. (For a more detailed look at walking, see Chapter 13.)

The problem with walking is that people tend initially not to do three things: they don't warm up or cool down properly; they don't allow for all weather conditions; and they don't walk tall. Weather conditions will affect anyone, but particularly those who have angina, with cold air causing pain.

Things you can do to help yourself:

- Dress properly, with layers of thin clothing, so you can take something off if you become too hot.
- Have a scarf with you – even in warm weather there can be a cold wind. Wrap a scarf around your mouth (only in really severe weather across the nose). Allow the natural air to pass in through your nose (warms it up before it reaches the lungs). Sit down if you get pain, take your spray or tablet, and take a few deep breaths.
- Walk tall. It is so easy when unwell or tired to curl our shoulders and stoop, but upright walking assists us not only to maintain bal-

ance, but to ensure that body weight is evenly distributed, thereby reducing uneven pressure and wear and tear on weight-bearing joints. Next time you pass a shop window and you notice your body is stooping, take a deep breath, lift both shoulders up to your ears as you do so, then circle them backwards and downwards as you breathe out. Immediately you will feel a lift in your body.
- Avoid activity after a heavy meal or eat smaller portions more often.
- If you smoke, stop (see Chapter 9).
- Instead of carrying heavy shopping bags, buy a shopping trolley (do not overload it) and shop more often.

One of my new participants came to the class because he kept experiencing pain in his chest on walking. It turned out that he did not warm up, started out at a quick pace, chose a route that was extremely hilly, and tended to shallow breathe. Exploration of the importance of warming up, starting slowly, building up the pace, occasional diaphragmatic breathing and slowing down near the end of the walk resulted in a significant change, which he excitedly told us about the very next week, stating that not only had he not had any pain or felt breathless, but he managed to get up the hill without stopping!

Other times to remember to deep breathe

When frustrated or feeling out of control

Taking a deep breath immediately calms us and gives us pause to think realistically about the situation, perhaps with a thought such as, 'I can control the way I feel. When I deep breathe I feel calmer.'

When seeing your doctor

Waiting for appointments naturally creates frustration because we want to be seen and helped quickly. But for some, the actual wait raises anxiety to such a level that their heart starts pounding. (See 'Seeing your doctor again' on page 17.)

Difficulty in sleeping

Sleep aids the recovery process, but is elusive for some. Deep breathing helps you to relax naturally (see the sleep guidelines on page 21).

Coughing

If you need to cough, place your hand across the scar tissue, and as you cough press gently with your hand (some people find a small cushion placed under the hand is helpful). Afterwards, take several deep breaths to ease the chest wall. Do the same for sneezing.

Injections

If you are concerned when having injections or blood taken, try telling the phlebotomist, 'I'm going to close my eyes, you just do what you need to.' Close your eyes, take several deep breaths, and concentrate on somewhere you love to be, take yourself there, deep breathe every now and again, and enjoy yourself.

If you are giving the injection to yourself, have it ready and place it against the skin. Take a deep breath and, as you breathe out, inject yourself. The out breath relaxes the body, stops discomfort and reduces soreness.

If you are suffering from constipation

This is common when you first take medication or after surgery, where inactivity inhibits the natural working of our system. Ensure you drink plenty of water, and use the breathing technique in the following way.

When your body feels the natural sensation that says you need to go to the toilet, take a deep breath and, as you breathe out, push down; this relaxes the muscles and eases the passage of your motion.

If after practising any of the above techniques you still suffer with any breathing difficulties, talk to your doctor to explore any possible underlying physiological problems.

6
Power of the mind as a healer

As already discussed, the mind is a powerful tool that can help or hinder the healing process because 'the way we think' ultimately affects 'the way we feel'. Remember that your thoughts may boost the release of serotonin (a natural feel-good chemical made by the body) or noradrenaline and cortisol, both known to lead to stress.

In this chapter I'm going to explain how you can help your recovery along with what I call *health-enhancing thoughts* – and how you can prevent the *health-inhibiting thoughts* that may hold your health back.

Let us first review the terms I will be using (Palmer and Tubbs, 2002):

- *Health-inhibiting thought (hit)* leading to *health-inhibiting beliefs (hibs)*.
- *Health-enhancing thought (het)* leading to *health-enhancing beliefs (hebs)*.
- Behaviours that fuel *health-inhibiting practices (hips)*.
- Behavioural change that fuels *health-enhancing practices (heps)*.

We are creatures of habit. Once a pattern of negative unrealistic or irrational thoughts is established, these thoughts can become absolutes, which fuel health-inhibiting beliefs and practices, leading into a downward spiral of distress. For example:

Health-inhibiting thought (hit): 'I can't do it' or 'I can't cope with this pain.'

This leads to:

Health-inhibiting belief (hib): 'I'm never going to cope with this pain.'

Conversely, look at the power of realistic positive thought:

Health-enhancing thought (het): 'This pain is bad, but when I make myself walk it eases.'

This leads to:

Health-enhancing belief (heb): 'I can help myself to reduce the pain.'

Unrealistic expectations of yourself and others

High demands on yourself and others can usually be traced back to stress-inducing beliefs such as:

- 'I should always put the needs of others first.'
- 'I ought to be seen to be able to cope well.'
- 'I have to get this job done before I take a break.'
- 'I must get this right, it's got to be perfect.'
- 'Other people ought to treat me fairly.'
- 'Other people must not upset me or behave in that way.'
- 'They have to help me, it's their job.'

And, these unrealistic expectations often fuel health-related beliefs such as:

- 'They'll be able to cure me, it's their job. The doctor will know what to do.'
- 'I've got to see the experts, only they can help me.'
- 'I can't stop smoking now, I've done it for too long.'
- 'I'm too long in the tooth to change now.'
- 'I can't change my diet, I'm far too busy. I haven't got the will power or time.'

Can you see how these demands create stress and wind up that 'internal spring'? (They also encourage a tendency to find excuses not to help yourself!)

What can you do to challenge such beliefs?

Look for the evidence that supports the belief

Ask yourself, 'Where is it written in any law book that I must, should, have too, or ought too?' It isn't, is it? Therefore if you constantly make such demands on yourself, you're just increasing your emotional discomfort.

Think of a hammer

I believe we all have an 'invisible hammer', and each time we get annoyed with ourselves or indeed others, we beat ourselves up with it. Most of the time my hammer has got a sponge on it. What's yours like, a battering ram perhaps?

Paul

Paul said, 'I use this hammer image all the time, especially when something's not going right. I just keep hammering away, and it doesn't help – it just makes it worse. But now, after working on it, whenever I start to get annoyed, telling myself I must sort this out, I just say sharply, "Enough, put the hammer down." It immediately makes me re-think.'

Review your preferences

We all naturally have a 'preference' for some aspect of our lives to be different, but if we constantly demand that it absolutely *should be*, *has to be*, *ought to be*, or *must not be so*, all we do is upset ourselves and make the situation worse.

Try using the word *prefer* instead of *must* or *ought*. It makes life much more comfortable and manageable.

Using hets to cope with unrealistic demands

Let's go back to the terms I reviewed at the start of this chapter: a *het*, or health-enhancing thought, can be used to challenge a *hit*, which is a health-inhibiting thought, leading to more positive and healthy behaviour. For example:

Hit: 'Oh no, I should have done that work.'
Replace with a het: 'There are no "shoulds". I would have preferred to have done it, but I haven't. Beating myself up won't get it done, so why not simply get on with it or leave it?'

This leads to:
Heb: 'I now believe I have more freedom in my choices and feel more relaxed.'

Write things down

It helps to write down any health-inhibiting thoughts and beliefs (*hits/hibs*) and then to write down contrasting health-enhancing thoughts and beliefs (*hets/hebs*). Sometimes people find it useful to grade each sentence in severity from 1 to 10, with 10 being the worst. Look at the following examples to see if you can identify with any of them (grade them for yourself):

Hit: 'Sitting here wallowing in self-pity isn't going to get the jobs done' (10).
(*Het/heb*): 'Being unwell is frustrating, but I can help myself to recover if I accept that getting better takes time' (6).

(*Hit*): 'I should be looking after others, not having them look after me' (9).
(*Het/heb*): 'I like to help others, but it is important to ensure I have the energy to do so by prioritizing my needs first' (5).

(*Hit*): 'I just can't cope with anything' (10).
(*Het/heb*): 'I'm coping with this illness just by choosing to use the medicine to help my body to heal. As long as I believe I am coping, I am' (6).

(*Hit/hib*): 'I have to get this right' (10).
(*Het/heb*): 'I know that I want to give my best to anything I do, but sometimes I'm not at my best, so whatever I do is good enough for that day' (4).

(*Hit/hib*): 'Only the doctors can help me to recover' (8).
(*Het/heb*): 'I believe that if I see the expert they will be able to help me, but I can also help by ensuring that I have a list of questions ready to ask and a pen to write down the answers' (2).

'I can't stand it!'

In a person with a heart condition (*and* without one!) this belief fuels continuing physical and mental distress, and may even increase pain. So how can you cope with low frustration tolerance that may also affect your recovery? Here's a story from my own experience:

After a visit to Disney World with long periods spent queuing, I recognized my extremely low tolerance to queuing! Upon returning from the trip, I reviewed my material and chose an exercise known as a 'shame-attacking' exercise. This means choosing to do something you normally find intolerable. Like most of you, I do not enjoy role play, but needs must, so I decided that as I cannot stand loud music I would play it in my car. As I switched the radio on my heart pounded at the thought of my elderly neighbours. Then a police car came towards me and I thought 'Oh no' – but they totally ignored me! I made myself drive down four high streets and eventually turned the engine off with relief, but also with wonderful clarity. It was as if a light bulb had come on in my head. Although I believed I could not stand loud music, the fact is I *could*: I'd just stood it for 35 minutes.

Now whenever I think 'I can't stand' something, I challenge it: 'Yes, you can, you *are* standing it, you've stood it for five minutes, and you can stand it for five more', showing that I *can* control the way I feel. Using it with the preference and breathing techniques, I now find I can tolerate most frustrating situations.

Identify when you feel frustrated

Is it when you go for a check-up, in a queue (my own bugbear), when driving, waiting for an appointment, being late or others arriving late?

How can you help yourself?

For example, waiting for an appointment. While you definitely have a preference to be seen at your scheduled time, demanding that you *should* be seen on time only leads to frustration, and probably a rise in your blood pressure. Try these thoughts instead:

'I have a right to be annoyed when my appointment is delayed, but I only upset myself by demanding I should be seen on time. I definitely would prefer to be seen punctually, but I can stand waiting, I've stood it before, and I can stand it again. I'll take a deep breath and read the paper.'

If you like this approach, try it out until you find a sentence that works for you, then write it down in your 'Coaching Myself to Health Book' and read it whenever you feel frustrated.

Feeling out of control

Because of your condition, you may feel out of control at times. This is a natural consequence of illness – our energy levels are sapped and we may have a tendency to see the worst in any situation ('awfulizing'). You may also feel controlled by your treatment. But *are* you?

Let's review the facts of a thought process known as *choices* – my personal favourite technique as it can work instantly. But everyone is different, and so if you don't find it helpful, just move on and try another technique instead.

Choices

I believe that, fundamentally, every single thing I do in this life, 'I choose to'. Even if someone has a gun and threatens to shoot me, while I accept they have fuelled the trauma with their behaviour, I still believe I have an element of choice.

However, every choice does have a consequence, which is why some people have problems with this process. You cannot accept choices unless you also accept the consequences of such a choice.

Some examples follow:

Having treatment of any kind

'Why have I got to have this treatment? I hate it!'
My choice: 'I haven't got to have it. I can say no and they won't give it to me. I am letting them give it to me, and it is my choice, because I'm choosing to want to get better.'

Taking medication of any kind

'This medication makes me feel sick, but I've no choice but to take it.'
My choice: 'I can choose not to take it, but then my illness could get worse. So I can choose to tell the doctor how it affects me and ask for a replacement, or ways to alleviate the problems. I'm in control when I do this.'

This invaluable tool of choice helps people to desensitize any emotional and physical effects created by self-defeating thoughts and beliefs that can intensify physical difficulties.

One woman believed she had no choice relating to 'pummelling'(her word for physiotherapy) and said she felt out of control with regard to this. We reviewed her choices, and over a period of time she recognized that everything she did she 'chose to'. Eventually she was able to feel more in control of her life, rather than controlled by the need for physiotherapy; as a result she needed less ‘pummelling’, and enjoyed improved health, increased independence, and fewer hospital visits.

7

Imagery as a healer

Imagery as a 'healer' is a very effective recovery tool, especially in lifting feelings of hopelessness or helplessness. Healing imagery encourages a person to believe in her ability to help herself, not only to feel better, but to help the immune system to work more effectively.

While imagery may appear to be most effective in relaxation, it is also a powerful tool in helping to:

- Cope with life's difficulties.
- Prioritize time to go to a 'safe' or 'favourite' place.
- Rehearse an expected or feared scenario.
- Evoke memories of lost loved ones.
- Encourage self-healing.
- Reduce the consequences of stress.

However, only 80 per cent of people 'see' in images. The other 20 per cent use their sense of smell, hearing, touch, taste or thoughts. So, first check if you are able to 'see' in images. Read the following script and then close your eyes. Take your time, and try to imagine the scene:

> Think of somewhere that is a special place for you, somewhere you love to be. Can you see it, can you feel it, or do you just know it is there? Open your eyes. Could you see it? Could you feel it? Or did you just know it was there?

If you cannot see in images, don't try to force yourself to do so; just allow the scripted words, or your other senses, to enjoy the body's relaxed state.

Contraindications to imagery

If you find you can only focus on a negative image (usually related to feeling severely depressed), do not, at this time, try out the imagery. Once your mood has lifted, practising the healing imagery will be beneficial. Ensure that your image does not include a picture of any fears you may have, such as heights, or if you are someone who is injury or blood phobic and may faint, make sure you are sitting down when you practise this.

Creating your own image to assist your recovery

Think for a moment and then write down:

- Where the pain or discomfort is felt.
- The level of pain or discomfort you have now (note the severity on a scale of 1 to 10).
- Any health-inhibiting thoughts that are generated when you think of the disease.
- How you see the disease now.
- How you would like to see it change.

Now think of an image you like that would help to combat any particular features of the way you feel.

John

John noted that his pain was spasmodic and mainly in his chest, but when it occurred it felt bad on a scale of 9/10 and he would be thinking, 'Oh no, I can't stand this pain.' He saw it like a vice tightening all the time, and wanted to see it unwind, releasing his chest. I created the following script for him:

John's healing imagery script (dots mean pauses):

Taking as many deep breaths as you like, each time you breathe out feel your whole body soften...Feel your ankles...your calves....your knees...your thighs soften...

Feel your buttocks, back, shoulders, elbows, wrists and your hands sink down...

Allow your head to rest gently on your shoulders...your eyes to soften...your lips to part slightly and the tongue to nestle in the lower part of the jaw...

As you breathe in, see that wonderful oxygen pass down towards your chest, blowing against the vice, cooling and soothing its grip...as you breathe out, any pain floats out and away from the body...

Every breath prises open the vice until you feel the chest rising and sinking effortlessly and the pain subsides. Say to yourself in your mind, 'As I breathe in my body relaxes, enabling me to help the healing take place. I am helping my chest to heal, I feel good, I feel content'...

Margaret

Margaret imagined a river almost blocked with rocks in order to describe the inside of her veins, saying, 'Some of them are huge, squeezing my blood into narrow streams, that seem to dribble in places.' She chose an image of a laser blaster carried into the body as she breathed in, taken to the area of blockage, releasing its powerful rays to blast away the rocks into tiny particles that were easily washed away whenever she passed water.

Other healing images

- Deep soothing breaths to unwind any spring (tension).
- A healing metaphor, e.g. a white light that penetrates any diseased area.
- A fighting metaphor, e.g. white blood cells like soldiers with bayonets attacking diseased cells, or oxygen pushing out the disease from the cells and releasing this waste through the normal excreting channels in the body.

Jean

Jean could not see things in images, but when asked to describe something she perceived as defensive and supportive, she immediately suggested a brick wall. We created a written script describing this wall and she also took a photo of her wall at home. At various times during the day she would look at the photo, close her eyes, say the words she liked in her mind, and see it protecting her from the illness that was invading her body.

The most important element of such practice is belief, belief that you can help yourself. It takes only a few minutes, but once it has been practised, it can easily become part of your everyday routine. Eventually you can create this image at any time, anywhere, within seconds.

If you like this approach to healing, you would benefit from reading a book called *Getting Well Again* by Simonton, Simonton and Creighton (see Further Reading).

8

Personal and work issues

This chapter looks at personal, relationship and work concerns that have caused stress in your past, are still affecting you now, or have arisen since your condition was diagnosed.

Personal issues

Recovery will normally take at least three months, but most people I know agree that it takes the first year to turn the most effective preventative care techniques into healthy habits. Time is the healer, so support it by accepting your limitations, and the inevitable up and down emotions, with self-help strategies, the first being the need to rest.

Let's look at the most common recovery issues.

Memory lapses

Memory loss is a natural outcome of any surgery, linked to both the anaesthetic and anxiety. But while any memory loss is likely to be temporary, always share any concerns with your doctor.

Here are some suggestions:

- Try not to worry. Memory lapses are often fuelled by concerns about your ability to recover, and too much time to think, so that you over-analyse. If you get annoyed because you cannot remember something, this makes it even harder to remember.
- Be honest. Say, 'I've forgotten its name, but it will come to me in a minute', and describe the object instead.
- Food stimulates brain power. For example, a US study in 2004 involving 14,000 female nurses found that those who ate plenty of green vegetables in their sixties suffered less mental decline in their seventies. Aim to include cruciferous vegetables, such as broccoli and cauliflower, and leafy foods such as spinach in your diet because they contain antioxidants and B vitamins, believed to protect the brain. While a good diet naturally provides adequate memory-stimulating vitamins and minerals, a supplement can give that added boost. Some people have tried Omega 3 sup-

plements, and many of them report improved memory.

- Keep a pad and pen by your chair and jot down any particular thoughts that are important to remember.
- Research shows mind games such as chess, crosswords, word puzzles, Scrabble and card games (such as crib, bridge and whist), and pastimes such as puzzles, painting and drawing, all stimulate the mind. One word of caution though – in the early stages of recovery, do not expect your concentration levels to be maintained for long periods of time. If you get frustrated, take a deep breath and close your eyes. Try to see the word written in your mind, open your eyes to try to solve the problem again and, if you can't, leave it and go back to it another time. If you are incapacitated for a while, make sure you have some of the items mentioned above to hand, picking them up whenever you feel you have the energy. Practice is the key to keeping the mind 'fit', so use it on a daily basis. The more we challenge our brains and keep them active, the more interconnections they make, and the easier it becomes both to concentrate and remember.

Focusing on the future or the past instead of the present

Being ill gives us time to think. For some, this is a reflective, comforting and indeed healthy pursuit that provides the opportunity to look at lifestyle issues that need changing. For others, it is a time of constant negative reflection on past experiences and future expectations that hinders comfort in the here and now.

If you constantly dwell on the past and its negative memories, or worry about the future, you risk suffering from depression and anxiety. Both of these are hindrances to recovery. Let's review what you can do to challenge such practices.

Focusing on the future

What do I do? First, I acknowledge it is normal to daydream an unpleasant thought or image. When I do, I allow it to be, and then say: 'Right, that's a good one, but it hasn't happened yet. I'm here now, and I'm OK, so come on and get on with the washing-up.' Encouraging yourself to do a mundane task is a very good way of breaking into a persistent negative thought that is creating distress (this is known as a distraction technique).

> ***Jim***
> Jim found he had a tendency to think ahead when sitting around all day, and was plagued by thoughts about never being able to work again, being in a wheelchair, and having recurrent heart attacks. He recognized that he needed to do three things – first, to acknowledge that such fears are normal and are better aired than suppressed; second, to allow the emotion to exist and then release it (he wrote down his fears, tore the sheet up and binned it); and third, to challenge the thought or image with a realistic statement such as, 'I'm not in a wheelchair, I have not had a heart attack since the first one and I'm recovering now, sitting here and allowing my body to rest. Come on, read your book.'

Focusing on the past

We all have past experiences that we would rather had not happened. They are ingrained memories, but when we dwell on them we are implying that they are still happening in the present. But take a realistic look: how can they persist into the present? Now is different from then; haven't you given yourself a chance to learn from your mistakes? I certainly have. Try using a statement such as (I use this one): 'That was then, and it was awful, but would I let the same thing happen now? No, I wouldn't, I've learnt from it, and it's not happening now.'

You may believe that your past behaviours, such as smoking or poor diet, have led to your health problem, but this too can be challenged. If you are making changes to your life, such behaviours are no longer to be feared.

> ***Harry***
> Harry used this health-enhancing thought to deal with his constant health-inhibiting belief of not being able to stay a non-smoker: 'I smoked heavily in the past and can still see myself puffing away, but that was then. Now I know it is not good for me, I have stopped, and it's not doing the same harm to me now.'

Another problem is mourning for a past that you perceive to be better than the present. If you are dwelling on the past as 'wonderful' you are probably feeling 'I'll never be that good again'. Think again: you may well have appeared healthier in the past than now, but somewhere and somehow, your behaviour may have begun your susceptibility to illness. By focusing on the here and now, you can reassess whether your past lifestyle was really as healthy as you thought, and, more importantly, recognize exactly what you need to do now to be healthier in the future.

Judging ourselves too harshly

When we are down or unwell we tend to evaluate ourselves negatively, or even question our purpose in life. I call this a temporary 'loss of identity'. As recovery proceeds, such thoughts and feelings naturally subside and are replaced with realistic positives of what you can do next. However, focusing only on repetitive negative thoughts can lead to depression. If this is the case for you, or if you are a carer who perceives this in your partner or 'patient', ask for support from your coronary care clinic or nurse, or your GP, who may prescribe a short course of antidepressants. While many people refrain from using them, they are not addictive if used appropriately and can provide the support you need in the early stages of your recovery. Most doctors' surgeries also have a counselling provision attached to the surgery, though waiting lists unfortunately vary from six weeks to six months – though we all have access to emergency services. Of course there are always private practitioners, skilled at helping individuals to review elements in their lives that are causing depression. Do check that they have understanding of heart conditions, as this would be an added benefit within any counselling you undertake.

Cognitive Behaviour Therapy (CBT)

I'm obviously biased because, as well as being a physical education specialist, I am also a Cognitive Behavioural Therapist and Health Coach, but I believe CBT is an ideal therapy for those with depression related to their illness because of its holistic proactive self-help philosophy. I liken myself to 'the keeper of the keys' – having the skills to unlock an individual's internal doors, though it is up to the person whether they wish to enter and have a good 'clear out'. In essence, the control stays with *you*, but the therapist's skills show you constructive ways – just as I'm trying to do in this book – to understand, deal with and effectively choose to change aspects of your life that are fuelling your depression.

There are several ways you can re-evaluate where you are and where you want to be:

First, who are you? Take a piece of paper and draw the outline of the letter 'I', covering the whole page. Write down inside the 'I' everything you can remember about yourself, starting with your basic identities (brother; sister; son; daughter; uncle; aunt, etc.). Include skills that you have (can use a computer; work within a team; delegate; good problem-solver, cook, seamstress; can do DIY, ride a bike, etc.); personal qualities (good listener; creative; innovative; loving; caring; honest; funny, etc.). Finish with aspects of yourself that you do not like (intolerant; short fuse; lazy; selfish; bother too much about what others think, etc.). If you have difficulty doing this, get your partner or carer to help you to reflect on your life.

Once you have finished (there's no rush, you can complete it over several days, or do it straight away and just add things when you think of them), draw a new 'I' and take each word and make it into a sentence starting with the word 'I', for example:

'I am a brother'
'I can work well in a team'
'I am skilled plumber'
'I am a skilled manager'
'I am a caring person'
'I try to be patient, but sometimes I'm not'

Now review the evidence for any negative beliefs and explore ways to realistically change them, for example:

Health-inhibiting thought: 'It really matters to me if others think I'm useless'.

Health-enhancing thought: 'I do care what others think about me, but I'm trying to value myself for what I do, which is all right most of the time'.

Now read your whole list to yourself. How does it feel? Try reading it out loud – does it make any difference? Sometimes, hearing ourselves speak has a more powerful effect, like being a third person listening in. Ensure that during your recovery you read this factual 'self-affirmations list' every day, either at night before you go to bed or any time you are beginning to question your worth.

Unrealistic expectations of self or others

Most people expect something to be done sooner or better – either by themselves or others. Recovery after illness is one of those times where pressure may seem to be from both sides. Either you expect yourself to get back to normal too quickly, or others do. Yet it is unrealistic to expect to resume normal life and routines immediately after an illness. You need time. You can deal with such anxiety, and still get things done, by trying this 'prioritizing' technique:

How to prioritize

Make a list of all the things you think you need to do tomorrow. Just note them down, no order of priority. Now, next to each one, write an A, B, C, D or E.

A means it is absolutely essential and needs to be done today.
B means it is important, but could be left until tomorrow.
C means it is not important at this time (remembering that Cs can turn into As, so they need daily reviewing).
D means delegation, whereby you realistically allow others to support you, or you to support others' personal development through exploring unfamiliar tasks.
E means questioning what personal 'energizer' I have for today (self-prioritizing), which will provide the fuel to deal with pressure/workloads.

For example, Len had the following chores to do and was getting anxious that he wouldn't be able to do them all. He wrote his list out as follows:

Put the rubbish out	A
Change the beds	C
Take my medicine	A
Get my pension	A
Ring Albert	B
Weed the front garden	B
Mend the light switch	B

Go for my recommended walk A

As you can see, his tasks immediately appear visually less, because only the As are essential. Len immediately felt less stressed. I then asked him to re-grade his As by numbering them in priority order:

Put the rubbish out A2
Take my medicine A1
Get my pension A4
Go for my recommended walk A3

Supposing you were Len and only managed to take your medicine before you felt unwell and couldn't do anything else. How would you feel? I suspect you might be thinking, 'Oh no, I haven't got the jobs done'. I would be thinking, 'Oh good, at least I got that one done'. Which of us would be more realistic – the one who focuses on what is not done, or the one who focuses on what has been done?

What time of day do you have the most energy – mornings, afternoons or evenings? I guess at the moment it will be mornings or afternoons. Therefore this is the time to deal with your main A1.

Len was living on his own so delegation was difficult, but we did look at how he could delegate some tasks to his children, particularly while he was recovering from his operation. He decided to ask his daughter to weed the front garden and his son to change his bedding next time they visited.

E for energy

The E element of this process is necessary to ensure you restore internal energy. In Len's example this would have been the walk.

Energy is something you probably feel very lacking in, so ensuring that your list of tasks includes an E for energizing is essential. To help you recognize when your energy levels are low, use images to help – perhaps a battery that needs recharging or the thermometer example given below. Remember if you cannot manage to 'see' in images, just allow the words to create understanding.

Imagine one of the old bulbous thermometers were inside you, with the bulbous part around the stomach area and the narrow part near the neck. When the thermometer is full, the dark line reaches up to the top and you feel full of energy. Every time you give that energy to someone else, it depletes your stock and the dark line goes down, leading to eventual exhaustion.

Does this happen to you? When and how often? Where? How does it feel?

A lot of men favour the image of the battery, linked with thoughts such as 'I need to recharge my battery' or 'I have just recharged my battery'.

If you cannot think of anything pleasurable or relaxing, look at your stability zones and rituals (see pages 41–2) and practise them. However, the most important E at the moment is rest and recuperation. This needs to be your E every day for a period in the morning and afternoon for the first few weeks after a heart attack and for three months after surgery.

When you have fully recovered you can use this prioritizing checklist for every major job in the house, breaking chores down into manageable chunks, and putting them in order of priority. As you complete each element of the task, tick it and say to yourself, 'Great! Well done.'

Tackling avoidance

Avoidance just stacks up problems and, when you don't feel well, adds to any feelings of incompetence. Facing a fear does the opposite: it always diminishes its effects.

- If you find a task on your prioritizing list that you keep putting down as a C and not dealing with it, mark the item with an asterisk. Make it a rule that when it gets to four asterisks, it becomes your A1 priority, and deal with it.
- Use the D for delegation. Give others the tasks that you are avoiding at this time, until you have fully recovered.
- If your avoidance is based on entrenched phobias, such as a fear of enclosed spaces, speak to your doctor who can refer you to a counsellor.
- Remember to encourage yourself to reflect on the present and what you can do now, rather than focusing on the past or future.

Work

Before your illness, was your job stressful, physically demanding, or mundane and boring? Do you now find yourself worrying about how you will cope with the work load or how your work is being covered by others? Are you concerned they may be doing it too well, or whether you will have a job to go back to? Do you fear that your employers are concerned that you will not be able to do your work efficiently or are not happy about you being off sick and therefore may sack you or make you redundant?

Any of these concerns stir up emotions that we might normally be able to shrug off. But when we have been ill, such concerns turn into fears that lead to us to undervaluing our skills, and doubting that others still want us.

Here are some suggestions:

1 Ensure that you discuss with your doctor how long you need to recuperate, which very much depends on the severity of the heart attack or surgery and their consequent physical effects on you. In my experience, sickness leave may range from two to eight weeks after a heart attack, and anything from three to six months after surgery. However, it is not just the doctor who needs to make this decision; *you* need to play an active part. Make sure you listen to your body and its messages, release emotions as already discussed, and ask yourself how you feel. Be frank with your doctor about this. Going back too soon and then needing more time off will only depress you.

2 As soon as you know how much time your recovery is expected to take, let your employers know and provide them with a formal sick note. Tell them that you will contact them (make a firm time and date) during the final week when you are off sick. This usually ensures that they leave you alone for the remainder of your recovery time and cuts the likelihood of you feeling pressurized (and in some cases bullied) to return sooner than you feel ready. If you feel unable to contact them yourself, make sure that a family member or carer does.

3 You will not help yourself or your work commitments if you keep phoning in to see how things are. Much as we hate to admit that we are all replaceable, the reality is that while others may not do

the job as well as us, they will at least be making the effort. If you think that's not good enough, you clearly have 'perfectionist' beliefs which might well have been one of the main factors in the development of your illness. However, peace of mind is important, so if you really are worrying and it is affecting your recovery, phone one colleague at work that you trust and share your concerns.

4 If you are not happy to return to work because it is too stressful, physically demanding, mundane or boring, ask yourself the following questions:

- Do I financially need to return to work and, if so, does it need to be to the same job?
- Do I need the same salary and, if not, how much can I afford to drop my income?
- Can I go part-time or job-share? After all, if my health is affected in the future, I won't be able to earn anything anyway.
- Can I take on light duties instead of heavy ones, or negotiate a staggered return?
- Is this the time to retire? If yes, can I negotiate early retirement?

Any of these negotiations can be started off by a letter or by an informal chat with a valued managerial or human resources colleague.

Talk to your family, share any thoughts and concerns, and listen to their views. Write out a 'for' and 'against' list for returning to work. Review financial commitments together, and which expenses can be reduced if you need to give up your job. At times we have all felt that we would love to retire and not work any more, but the reality can be quite scary. When I worked in adult education we ran courses on 'How to cope with retirement'. Many of the attendees were anxious about giving up work, fearing that their purpose in life would be lost. Make a list of all the things that you have enjoyed doing in your life (even if you are no longer doing them), plus any that you would like to try; if you have a partner, ask them to do the same. Read the 'interest/leisure' pages of the newspaper and ask friends who are retired what they do with their day. Sit back and carefully review your list; it provides a resource of recreational activities and experiences that can make retirement as fulfilling as working.

5 If you are happy to return to work, but worried about your ability to cope with the pressure, make sure that at the end of each day you write out your perceived work list for the next day and prioritize using the ABCDE process. I frequently use this process when working with people who suffer from work-related stress, who without exception report a reduction in their unrealistic expectations of themselves. By using this tool they also invariably find they get more work done, blame themselves far less for 'inefficiency' and, most importantly, suffer less overload and enjoy greater confidence.

Debbie

Debbie, when feeling under pressure, immediately 'ABCDE's' her list (the E, or energy restorer, is always her lunch break) and is able to desensitize her initial health-inhibiting thought (*hit*) of 'Oh, I've got so much to do' into a health-enhancing thought (*het*) of 'Well, only the As are essential, so I'll re-write them and number them in priority order. Only number 1 is absolutely essential – everything else is a bonus.'

If you find you are still focusing on the amount of tasks you can see on your list, re-write the As, Bs and Cs on to separate pages and place them under each other. At once, visually, you will see you have less to do. Once the As are clearly defined in importance, look and see if any can be Ds or delegated to someone else. If you are in a position of authority, delegate wherever possible. This will achieve two things. First, you will be giving someone opportunities to develop their skills, and second, you will lessen your workload and your stress, enabling you to concentrate on one aspect of your work, so releasing the guilt associated with doing too many jobs not as thoroughly as you would like.

6 Do you have a tendency to take on board other people's workload? Remember that your condition has probably been caused by a number of lifestyle factors, and if you believe that work stress is one of them, you need to reassess your behaviour. Using the prioritizing list has enabled many people who formerly took on board others' problems to re-evaluate. Rather than immediately

leaping at any extra work offered them, they have taken a moment to consider, saying, 'Just let me see what my priority today is, and if it's not as important as your problem, I'll help you with it.'

It's important to remember that you have a choice, because if you choose to take on others' problems, you need to accept the consequences – overload! Ask yourself whether you are actually helping someone if you continuously sort out their problems. How will they learn to cope for themselves? Show them the prioritizing ABCDE instead – who knows, it could be good for their long-term health too!

7 If you feel that work is stressful because you are being bullied, consider taking an assertiveness training course. This does not teach you to be aggressive, but provides you with the skills to help you stand up for yourself, leaving little chance for misunderstandings, while at the same time being sensitive and sympathetic to the needs, feelings and rights of other people. Assertiveness, properly used, creates respect and value for yourself and others, and may involve you saying 'no' and being honest, rather than saying 'yes' to please others.

8 If you have a tendency to work until you drop, or eat your lunch at your desk, your energy resources will quickly become depleted. Always have constructive breaks. I have proved to people many times that if you take a drink break in the morning and afternoon, and a full lunch break, you actually end up completing more work. Most importantly, you do not want work stress to exacerbate factors that have already affected your health. There follow some tips to help you re-fuel your energy and concentration levels.

Some work-related tips

- When you are tired, stop what you are doing. Take a deep breath while raising your shoulders up towards your ears, and circle them backwards and downwards as you breathe out. If you have stiffness in your fingers, circle your hands four times one way and four times the other, and open and close your fingers into a fist four times (increases circulation and reduces tension).
- As you begin your break, take two deep breaths, circle your shoulders etc. as before, and stand up. If you work in a building

with stairs, walk down the stairs to the bottom (maximum of six flights down). Comfortably deep breathe as you do so. The return journey up is always slower as it is harder to climb! If you are still in the early stages of recovery, begin with two flights of stairs down and up and increase slowly. On returning to your office, make yourself a drink and sit down, but do not start working until you have finished your drink.

- Assess which is your best time of the day. If it is the morning, make the afternoon break five minutes longer, or vice versa.
- Wherever possible, ensure you take your lunch break (a minimum of half an hour), preferably away from the office. If you have nowhere to go, ensure you take a good book or magazine to work and sit away from the hustle and bustle.
- If your work was the mainstay of your life and you cut down on leisure pursuits or time with your partner, now is the time to make changes. Make a time list in your diary or on a board at home (such as the one shown in Table 8.1) and maintain it daily.

Table 8.1 Example of a time list

Time for work	*Time for leisure*	*Time alone with my partner*	*Time to socialize*	*Time for self*	*Time with my family*	*Time for exercise*	*Time to relax*

Under each section, note down the time you expect to, or wish to, spend on that particular aspect, ensuring that there is time at least once a day for one activity that gives you pleasure. (Remember, E is for energizer.)

9

How to give up smoking

I know that most of you reading this book will have been advised to give up smoking and that many of you have already done so, but there are a few who still stick to the belief 'I *can't* give up'. I have researched and compiled this next section to help you to face the reality of continuing to smoke; if then you decide to continue, the consequences are all yours. Just remember that smokers are twice as likely to suffer recurrent heart attacks or strokes as non-smokers because nicotine raises blood pressure and carbon monoxide joins on to the red pigment of the blood and reduces its power to carry oxygen to the heart and all other parts of the body.

In fact, of the 120,000 who die because of smoking each year in the UK (one-fifth of all deaths), around 30,000 are victims of cardiovascular disease. Some 1,000 young people die of heart disease related to smoking each year.

If you smoke, you are putting the following inside your body:

- 4,000 chemicals, tar and carbon monoxide.
- Acetone – a solvent found in nail polish remover.
- Ammonia – found in strong cleaning fluids.
- Arsenic – a poison used in insecticides.
- Benzene – used as a solvent in fuel and in chemical manufacture.
- Cadmium – a poison used in batteries.
- Formaldehyde – a poison used to preserve dead bodies.
- Hydrogen cyanide – an industrial pollutant.

Having said all this, I know that giving up is not easy. There are three aspects to overcome. First, the actual physical addiction to nicotine; second, the habit part; and third, the psychological change that needs to happen in order to maintain the no-smoking regime. Remember that just one year after quitting smoking you halve your chances of worsening your heart condition.

Even if you have been smoking for a long time, giving up has its benefits because as soon as you give up, the risk of a second heart attack is reduced.

In the short term:

- Just 20 minutes after you stop smoking, blood pressure and pulse return to normal, and circulation to hands and feet improves.
- Eight hours after you stop, the oxygen level in your blood increases to a normal level, and the chances of a heart attack start to fall.

In the long term:

- From the moment you stop smoking, the risk of a heart attack starts to reduce and is halved after one year of stopping smoking.

Aids to stop you smoking

To help yourself to make and maintain this life-changing decision, you first need to be prepared for the inevitable daily withdrawal symptoms from both the nicotine and the emotional crutch of having a cigarette in your hand. Once you're clear of these, the most important move is to search out support networks and leaflets that give you constructive tools to stop and stay stopped.

- The NHS has a stop smoking helpline and most doctors' surgeries or health clinics now run 'stop smoking clinics' which may offer one-to-one discussions with trained advisers, and help with the cost through bulk prescriptions or, if you are on benefits or receiving family credits, free prescriptions.
- Many treatments are available including NRT (Nicotine Replacement Therapy) in the form of:
  - Gum: absorbed through the lining of the mouth as you chew.
  - Lozenges: similar to a sweet that you suck slowly.
  - Patches: give a constant supply of nicotine and are available for 12, 16 or 24 hours' duration.
  - Micro tabs: a tablet dissolved on the tongue.
  - Nasal spray: dissolved through the lining of the nose, and good for extreme withdrawal symptoms.
  - Inhalator: similar in shape to a cigarette, a nicotine cartridge fits in to the top and releases the nicotine as and when it is needed. Helpful if you miss the hand-to-mouth action of smoking.

Other ways of stopping smoking/coping strategies

Zyban

This is not Nicotine Replacement Therapy, but is often used alongside more traditional methods. It is only available on prescription. It is a tablet that is taken daily, normally over a period of between seven and nine weeks.

'Cold turkey'

This means you decide never to have another cigarette and do not smoke at all.

Cutting down

This is a lengthy process, and one that needs a determined mind. Decide on a date and a time when you will stop completely. Then aim to reduce your smoking by one cigarette a day, e.g. 20 cigarettes a day. Reducing by one a day would take you three weeks to stop (40 = 6 weeks and so on). Write down the date, and get a friend or family member to witness your signature. Each day write on your cigarette packet how many cigarettes you are allowed and take out any surplus.

Using a diary

Use a diary and write down for one week the times and places in a day that you smoke a cigarette, how important it is to you, and what rating you give it from 1 to 5, with 1 being low, and 5 being high.

Make a list showing your least and most needed cigarettes. Start by cutting out the cigarettes that you rated as 1, the next week those that were 2, etc. until you reach the most difficult number, 5, by which time your desire will have decreased and you are more likely to be able to give up.

Time limits

Some people find it easier to give up if they set time limits, e.g. smoking one cigarette every hour, and then increasing the time each week by half an hour until they reach a point where they are only smoking two a day. They can then give up one the following week, and one the week after.

Set boundaries with smoking

DO NOT:

- Smoke in the bedroom, and slowly ban it from other areas of your home until it becomes smoke free.
- Smoke as soon as you get up. Smoking before breakfast irritates the lining of the stomach, making you more likely to develop a peptic ulcer.
- Smoke just before you go to bed.
- Smoke during a meal or an hour before it. Smoking suppresses the appetite.

DO:

- Sit in a no-smoking area while travelling or when eating a meal.
- Keep active. Inactivity leads to boredom and an increased desire to smoke.
- Throw away anything that is associated with smoking.
- Take four deep breaths and actively distract yourself whenever the urge to smoke feels greatest.
- Go to the dentist and have your teeth cleaned and polished.
- Put the money you would normally spend on cigarettes in a jar and treat yourself in some way.
- Let others know you have given up and ask them not to smoke in front of you.
- Write down all the positive things you have noticed since you stopped smoking such as: easier breathing, more stamina, cleaner teeth, better sense of smell and taste, fresher smelling clothes and hair, and a feeling of tremendous achievement.
- Use family friends to be around at times that are 'high risk'.
- Support your family by banning smoking from your house. Remember that passive smoking is still dangerous, and more so when you have a condition that affects the heart.

Power of the mind

As with any addictive habit, we can always find reasons why now is not a good time to give up. Even when we decide to, complacency can quickly take over, and as the mental addiction is as strong as the physical addiction, our brain can trick us into starting again before we even know it by releasing thoughts such as 'I can just have one when I go out socially' or 'I'll just have a couple a week' or 'I'm not smoking as much as I was, so that's still good'.

Feelings of failure are common among people who are trying to quit any habit. The most important thing is not to stop quitting. You need to remind yourself why you wanted to stop, what you have achieved so far, and to remember that change is better maintained when it is slow and progressive.

One of the most powerful tools to help suppress cravings is the way we think, using realistic positive thoughts, beliefs and behaviours such as:

Health-enhancing thoughts:
'I can do it. I've managed to leave it for a few hours, so I can time myself and make it longer between cigarettes.'

'I've got nicotine inside me that's been there a long time. I need to give myself time, and I can keep plugging away. I can do it because I want to.'

This leads to health-enhancing beliefs:
'I managed it yesterday; it was tough, but I'll keep using the patches and the deep breathing. I'm doing well.'

This leads to health-enhancing practices:
'I'm taking one day at a time. Each morning I read my thoughts' script and remind myself how well I am doing and then I put a new patch on.'

Coping with the cravings

When you first stop smoking your body reacts with withdrawal symptoms. Table 9.1 lists some of the most common withdrawal symptoms and gives suggestions on how to deal with them:

Table 9.1 Common withdrawal symptoms when you give up smoking

Symptoms	*How it feels/the cause*	*How to cope*
Cravings	An intense desire to smoke. This will reduce over a few weeks	Do something different to distract yourself. Take a few slow deep breaths. Drink a glass of water. Use NRT. Cravings normally pass in 3–5 minutes
Coughing/dry mouth	This is caused by the lungs clearing out the tar	Warm drinks can ease the cough. Coughing shows the lungs are recovering
Hunger	This is caused by the change in your metabolism	Keep healthy snacks like fruit and vegetables to hand. Try chewing gum and drink lots of water
Bowel changes	Possible constipation and diarrhoea	It will settle. Drink lots of fluids and include more fibre if constipated
Trouble sleeping	As the nicotine leaves the body, you may experience tiredness	This settles after the first 2–3 weeks; more exercise and less tea and coffee will help
Dizziness	Caused as more oxygen instead of carbon dioxide reaches the brain	This will pass on its own after a few days
Mood swings, irritability, unable to concentrate	Caused by the withdrawal of nicotine and missing the habit of smoking	Turn to friends or family for support; use coping methods

Stress management

Every time you get an urge to smoke, take five to ten deep breaths and think, 'I don't need that cigarette, I feel better now I've had a deep breath, more relaxed.'

Write down your feelings when you crave a cigarette. Really let rip! Read it only once, then tear the paper into tiny pieces and throw it into the bin. Now sit down and make a list of the benefits you have achieved so far from not smoking and praise yourself.

We tend to depend on smoking when feeling stressed or when we are in social situations, especially if we are around other smokers. Anticipating these situations and preparing to deal with them in a positive way is very important. Prepare yourself before you go out by using 'rehearsal imagery'. Close your eyes and picture yourself entering the social event, see yourself looking well, smiling and chatting to others. When you see people smoke, hear yourself say, 'Everyone is turning away as they puff. That was me before, but not now. I'm healthier, and everyone is happily chatting to me. I can cope with not smoking, and indeed I am coping. I see myself take a deep breath when I want to smoke. I've just realized I've been talking for over an hour and I haven't even thought about a cigarette. Well done! You're doing it.'

Write out a list of sentences giving health-enhancing thoughts and beliefs and put them into your 'Coaching Myself to Health Book'. Read them whenever you feel like giving up your goal of not smoking.

Table 9.2 lists some common triggers of the craving to smoke, and ways of dealing with them.

However, even the strongest resolve can be broken at times. Many people who give up smoking suffer a relapse, and it is at this time that we need to be at our strongest. It is important to:

- Stop smoking again immediately (if you need more help, go back to your doctor).
- Recognize the reasons why you felt the need to smoke and gave in to the temptation. Write them down so that next time you will know what to expect and have a better chance of getting over that hurdle.
- Remind yourself that you have achieved a great deal in trying to give up and that the result will be to your benefit.

- Ask friends and family to support you in the difficult times and remember that if you really want to give up you will succeed.

(See Useful addresses for extra help and support.)

Table 9.2 Some common triggers in smoking and ways of dealing with them.

Trigger	*How to deal with it*
Getting bad news	*Think* – Smoking will not change the bad news, nor will it cure any problems
	Do – Have a good cry and talk to a friend
After an argument	*Think* – I can cope with this situation without smoking
	Do – Get away from the problem for a few minutes, and take deep breaths and relax
Being with smokers	*Think* – Deep down they wish they could quit too
	Do – Smile, think NOPE (Not One Puff Even)
Feeling happy	*Think* – I can celebrate without a cigarette
	Do – Treat yourself, sing, dance, laugh
Having a drink	*Think* – I can learn to enjoy a drink without smoking
	Do – Keep your hands busy

10

Cutting down on alcohol

Moderate drinking (between one and two units of alcohol a day) is thought to help protect the heart in men aged over 40 and post-menopausal women, although you should have at least one or two alcohol-free days per week.

Drinking to excess is now becoming an epidemic, with 1 in 25 people being dependent on alcohol. This can damage the heart muscle, increase blood pressure and lead to weight gain. If you feel you need to reduce your alcohol intake, read on.

Support for chronic drinkers

Compared with the support available to smokers and drug addicts, there is less help for alcoholics or high-alcohol consumers, but let's review what there is. One of the most powerful tools in stimulating cravings is related to the way we think, such as:

Health-inhibiting thought: 'I can't cope without a drink.'

This leads to the *health-inhibiting belief*: 'I need to drink – it takes my stress away.'

This leads to the *health-inhibiting practice*: 'Refill my glass.'

Conversely, the power of the mind can be used to suppress the desire as in the *health-enhancing thought*: 'When I drink I end up feeling more stressed not less.'

This leads to *health-enhancing beliefs*: 'I know that I am drinking just to feel better; it works for the first drink, and then I start to feel down, and I want to obliterate everything. I need to find other ways to deal with this stress and then I can enjoy a drink.'

This leads to *health-enhancing practices*: 'I'm not going to the pub at lunchtime. I'm going to bring in a sandwich and stay in the office, or go out with a colleague to the café.'

Points to bear in mind with regard to alcohol intake

- Be aware of the recommended safe alcohol intake, i.e. 3–4 units a day for men and 2–3 units a day for women; 1 unit is half a pint of lager, 1 measure of spirit, or 1 small glass of wine.
- Keep a diary for a month and note down where, when, how frequently and how much you drink. Is there a pattern fuelled by social life, work, or stress at home?

Use the information in the following ways:

- Reduce intake by having smaller glasses or drinking halves.
- Have a glass of water in between each alcoholic drink (very helpful with wine drinkers, especially if the water is in a wine glass).
- Have non-alcoholic drinks.
- Drink from a glass, not a bottle.
- Sip slowly rather than gulp.
- Have shandies, with diet lemonade, rather than full pints of beer.
- Try to eat before or while you are drinking, as food delays the absorption of alcohol into the body.
- Don't visit pubs or wine bars in your lunch hour (makes you more lethargic, affects concentration and causes mood swings; and the smell of alcohol often offends colleagues, leading to alienation).
- Speak to your doctor or find and use alcohol advisers who are sometimes based in health clinics.
- Use alcohol counsellors or attend groups for alcohol abusers.
- If you use alcohol as a way of releasing stress, explore the benefits of health coaching; counselling – particularly cognitive/behavioural and the therapy known as 'rebt'; stress management and alternative therapies, to change behavioural habits that fuel the desire to drink, and so help you manage any stress in your life.
- Pellets can be implanted into the stomach and will make you sick if you drink alcohol (you must seek medical advice on this).
- Antabuse pills are available but not yet licensed; these are said to give a feeling of a bad hangover if you drink too much alcohol.
- A patch similar to that used by smokers is being considered to help curb excessive alcohol consumption.

Contact organizations that help alcohol users – see Useful addresses.

11

Developing healthy eating habits

Food is our 'living fuel', yet we tend to take it for granted – sometimes using it to reward ourselves for working hard, but most often to stifle feelings of boredom, loneliness and stress.

Our pace of life, high calorific eating habits fuelled by advertising, and the diversity of prepared food, linked with inactivity, have led to a tendency for the body to store enormous amounts of sugar and carbohydrates which clog the arteries and result in people being overweight or actually obese. I believe we have become 'acceptors' instead of 'selectors' of what is or what is not healthy eating.

An unhealthy diet affects the workings of the heart by not supplying essential vitamins and minerals, and an excess of saturated fats leads to a range of serious disorders such as diabetes and heart disease. An estimated 46 per cent of deaths from coronary heart disease are caused by too much cholesterol (BHF, 2004).

Many feel their diet has contributed to their developing coronary heart disease, but believe that change, often years after particular habits have formed, can be extremely difficult. Many naturally turn to various diets because they hold out the tantalizing prospect of a relatively easy, quick-fix solution. We want instant change; it appears easier to handle, but we really need time to implement our chosen changes. The problem is that these diets do not reflect the differing physical, emotional, mental and behavioural components of any one individual. What is right for one is not necessarily right for another. Use your time now to reflect and to make gradual changes, because change is better maintained when it is slow and progressive.

I'm sure you have read many food guidelines about healthy and unhealthy foods and some of these may seem confusing. One day it's all right to eat this, the next, watch out – it could lead to such-and-such a condition. This section is not about reflecting on the rights or wrongs of these debates, but on reviewing aspects of your diet that may have contributed to developing CHD, and exploring effective tools to maintain a healthy diet and, ultimately, improved health.

Benefits of healthy eating

- Keeps blood cholesterol levels low, reducing the likelihood of fatty material clogging up the arteries.
- Keeps blood pressure down by helping to prevent blood clots from forming.
- Reduces the likelihood of being overweight or having a stroke.
- Increases the chances of survival from a heart attack.

Healthy eating

Aim to have 'balance' – not too much of any one thing – through a diet that includes plenty of fruit, vegetables, starchy foods and moderate amounts of dairy products, meat, fish and other proteins.

Let's break down food into four simple groups:

1 Cereals, bread, pasta, rice and potatoes
2 Fruit and vegetables
3 Meat, poultry, fish, pulses, cheese, nuts and eggs
4 Dairy products

Foods from groups 1 and 2 should be the main part of each meal, with intake from groups 3 and 4 kept to smaller portions (preferably with fish eaten more often than red meat). You should also aim for five portions of fruit and vegetables per day.

A useful tool to encourage and recognize changes you are making is to write these intended changes down and keep them visible, either inside a cupboard or on a fridge door. For example:

To reduce fat I am – using skimmed milk
To reduce salt I am – using salt either in cooking or on the table
To reduce sugar I am – drinking tea and coffee without sugar
To increase fibre I am – using wholemeal bread instead of white

Healthy eating and drinking plan

- Aim to drink at least seven glasses of water a day, but no more than two glasses at night as the kidneys like a rest. Sip rather than gulp, to combat dehydration effectively. If you are drinking large amounts of water at night, tell your doctor, as this could be a sign of too much salt, sugar or alcohol in your diet.
- Avoid food and drinks that make your heart race. Cut down on fizzy drinks, or tea and coffee, and use decaffeinated coffee, herbal teas, low-calorie cola, or alternate tea with a cup of hot/cold water (works wonders for the digestive system). Green tea has been found to guard against cardiovascular disease because it lowers blood pressure, total cholesterol levels, and reduces platelet aggregation.
- Cut out or cut down on your weekly intake of cakes, sweets, processed foods, crisps, salty snacks, sandwiches and fast foods.
- Make vegetables and salads the main part of any meal except breakfast, which, in order to generate energy, needs to be high fibre; porridge is the best choice as it lowers cholesterol.
- Have at least two days when you do not eat meat and eat two portions of oily fish (not fried) a week.
- Eat five portions of fruit and vegetables daily (their antioxidant vitamins A, C and E increase the amount of blood circulating in the brain). If you are working or intend to return to work, take some raw vegetables to eat with your lunch and keep some in your fridge as snacks.
- Aim to eat brown rice instead of white, wholegrain cereals, bread and pasta, and reduce your intake of butter, cream and full-fat milk. Instead, choose low-fat yoghurt, polyunsaturated margarine, semi-skimmed or fully skimmed milk, low-fat cheese and yoghurt.
- Grill and bake instead of frying. Cutting off fat and skin from poultry before you cook will substantially reduce your intake of fat, which should not exceed 35 per cent of daily calories. Cook stews and soups slowly, skimming off any fat regularly.
- Wherever possible, use fresh foods rather than processed as they have a higher nutritional value and are free of added salt. However, it is better to use frozen vegetables rather than have none at all.
- Eat fresh fruit and vegetables as soon after purchasing as possible as the vitamin content will decrease with storage. Storing in a

refrigerator and reducing cooking time helps to lessen this loss.

- Gradually reduce the amount of salt you add to your food. Either add salt to cooking or have it on the table, never both. If you are buying tinned vegetables, ensure they are clearly marked 'no added salt'.
- Lastly, go shopping every day – it increases your exercise – but ensure that you buy only what you need for that day or, at the most, two days. Most importantly, read labels and buy foods that are higher in polyunsaturates and fibre (at first this takes time, but with practice you get quicker).

Heart-friendly foods

Try to include in your diet foods known to help combat coronary heart disease:

- A daily dose of sesame oil is said to help to lower blood pressure.
- Blueberries (a large handful) provide as many antioxidants as five servings of carrots, apples, broccoli and squash.
- A daily glass of pomegranate juice slows down cholesterol build-up and reduces blood pressure, doubling levels of health-boosting antioxidants in the blood.
- Potassium (found in bananas) lowers blood pressure.
- Almonds produce calcium, the bone-building mineral.
- Peanuts help the heart by boosting the B vitamin called folate.
- Hazelnuts are rich in vitamin E, which protects cell walls from damage by free radicals. The oil from hazelnuts is almost identical in nutritional composition to the heart-friendly olive oil.
- Walnuts are rich in a type of good fat called alpha linolenic acid; this has a specific blood-thinning and anti-clotting effect.

Losing weight

For those who feel the need to lose weight, or have been advised to do so, it can seem an insurmountable mountain to climb at the same time as trying to recover from coronary heart disease. My advice is *don't* think of it as a diet. Try to think of it as a life change, like switching to a new job or moving house. Naturally you may be nervous and uncertain, but with time and practice things really will become easier and turn out for the better.

For most of you, the dietary measures already discussed will naturally lead to weight loss, but sometimes further help is needed. There are also external influences that can help or hinder changes in eating habits:

Other members of the family

In a family, there may be a tendency to provide the everyday foods (and treats) that people are used to, providing constant temptation. Engage your family in the process of changing their eating habits too – involve them in choosing foods, or set them the task of finding alternatives to foods deemed to have a high cholesterol content. Children are very good at working out labels once they know the major 'no' aspect to look out for.

Stress

Too much stress fuels the desire to eat – we often understand the theory, but have difficulty in putting it into practice. We want comfort, and food provides it! If you feel this is the case, have a look at the tips on beating stress in Chapter 4.

Living alone

If you live alone, it can be easier to buy healthy foods because you can actually say no to yourself. But if you feel lonely, food is often the comforter. In this case, talk to your doctor, and ask a family member or friend to shop for you at first, with you eventually accompanying them to the shops. Make out a list of all the fruits and vegetables you already like and see if once a week you can try a new one, so slowly building up your 'portfolio' of healthy foods. Consider exploring the internet, which is a good provider of information on effective ways to eat healthily.

> ***Keith***
> Keith lived alone, and was becoming frustrated and anxious as the weeks went by and had received no follow-up appointment after diagnosis. After a great deal of *hits* (*health-inhibiting thoughts*, see Chapter 6), such as 'I can't cope with it on my own, they should be looking after me', during which he stayed in and was afraid to go out, he began to take more responsibility for his own health, using the internet to research information about healthy eating and his condition. To date, he has set up an exercise and eating programme that has reduced his weight by over 2

stone, and feels both healthier and happier – all this before he was even seen at the clinic.

Three golden rules in dieting

Essentially, there are three main aspects to successful dieting:

1 Wanting to, and believing you can do it.
2 Not beating yourself up if you go off track, but starting again immediately.
3 Praising yourself at the end of each day for anything you have succeeded in maintaining.

Supporting yourself as you change your diet

- Aim to eat at least three moderate-sized meals rather than one large meal as our metabolism works more efficiently when given a steady supply of food.
- Gradual reduction/change is far more effective at reducing withdrawal symptoms (see Table 11.1).

Table 11.1 Ways of changing your diet

Past practice	*Change to*
Using butter in sandwiches, etc.	Reducing intake of butter, cream and full-fat milk, by only having them once a week. At all other times have low-fat yoghurt, polyunsaturated margarine, low-fat cheese, etc.
Skimmed milk	Semi-skimmed before attempting skimmed

If you have difficulty imagining the weight of a particular piece of food (which is my problem), try this simple visual process. See 3 oz of meat as the size of your palm, 2 oz of cheese as a pair of dominoes, a cup of vegetables as a clenched fist. Create other stimulating images for yourself. Weigh the items first and then think what they remind you of.

- Set a realistic target of weight loss, i.e. 1–2 lbs a week, 4 lbs a week if you are very overweight or obese. Remember that excess weight is more likely to stay off if it is a slow and consistent process.

- Don't persistently use scales – 'listen' to your body and look at it. After a month, try on an item of clothing that previously felt tight – how does it feel now?
- Make a list of foods that do not have a high calorific content, but still provide vitamins and minerals, such as: 1 oz of carrots, 7 calories; a heaped tablespoon of greens or potatoes (boiled), 6 and 20 calories respectively.
- Eat wholemeal bread, pasta, wholegrain cereals, brown rice and potatoes in their skins.
- Avoid eating shellfish more often than once or twice a month as it contains a cholesterol-like substance.
- Limit whole eggs to three per week, because the yolk is rich in cholesterol. However, you can eat as much egg white as you wish.
- Instead of mince, buy lean stewing beef and casserole it before mincing.
- Opt for low-calorie snacks such as sliced vegetables and keep them in the fridge; every time you feel like something sweet, have a piece of vegetable first as it will help to dampen cravings.
- Cut down on alcohol as it contains about 100 calories in a single unit. Ensure you have two alcohol-free days a week and no more than two drinks a day for men, and half that for women.
- A diet rich in fibre will encourage weight loss as it helps the bulk of food to break down and leave the body.

Keep a food diary

You need to assess your eating habits in order to effectively change them. Start by keeping a diary, noting down for two weeks all the food you eat; how much; what time of day; where you were; and what you were thinking before, during and after you had eaten. Through this diary you will see patterns emerge of healthy and unhealthy eating.

Mary

Mary's diary highlighted that whenever she couldn't sleep she would come downstairs and have something to eat, usually a biscuit, thinking, 'I'm exhausted, I'll never be able to work tomorrow, I need my sleep but I just can't get it; at least a biscuit makes me feel better.' This usually led to further biscuits and a cup of coffee. Eventually she would go back to bed and try to sleep, often waking in the morning with indigestion and extreme fatigue. She also found that her intake of sugary foods increased during the day, along with copious amounts of coffee.

It only takes 100 to 200 extra calories a day over a decade to make us obese, but starving yourself never works, because biologically the body reacts by slowing down its metabolism, thereby becoming used to working on fewer calories. If the dieter then reverts to an increased calorie intake, the extra calories join the fat store because the body's slowed-down metabolism no longer requires them.

Therefore a healthy balance between calorie intake and calorie burn is the only way to reduce and maintain a desired weight. In other words, output needs to be greater than input – hence the importance of exercise alongside a diet combined with a selection (in moderation) of all foods.

Tips to improve digestion and reduce an excessive intake of food

- Eat slowly, chew well and swallow fully before your next mouthful. The stomach will feel fuller and the desire to eat more will diminish. Eating quickly often results in indigestion, with bloated and tired feelings.
- Put your food on smaller plates.
- Avoid reading or watching television when eating. This represses responses, takes away the enjoyment and taste of the meal, and usually means you are eating faster.
- Be confident in your ability to take control.
- When eating out, have a light starter or none at all, ask for low-fat dressing, ensure your main meal has some vegetables with it, and have fruit for desert.
- If a glass of water is taken half an hour before a meal, it suppresses appetite.
- Aim to have your main meal before 7 p.m. (for those who work no later than 8 p.m.), as the digestive system slows down in the evening, and most residue food becomes stored as fat. Definitely no biscuits with coffee/tea before you go to bed – it inhibits sleep. There are two and a half teaspoons of sugar in a biscuit (that's plain ones).
- Whenever possible, make your midday meal your main one and have a snack for your tea, as this gives you time to burn off the calories before you go to bed.

- Take a deep breath just before you eat and in between each mouthful or at any time you feel the urge to eat calorie-rich food. Use a relaxation tape to distract and relax you. Relaxing will lessen the desire to eat, as adequate rest is an important factor in reducing stress and appetite.

Support when trying to lose weight

Some people find it very difficult to maintain a diet on their own. If this is the case with you, join a slimming club with a friend or involve your partner. Ensure you do not cut out vital nutrients and vitamins that you need for your recovery. Most importantly, if you go off track, don't give up; simply start again as soon as you can, or ask your doctor to refer you to a nutritionist.

In 2005 the British Dietetic Association planned a campaign, sponsored by Pfizer, aimed at encouraging people to lose weight sensibly and slowly. (You can phone 0800 056 8695 to receive a free booklet on cholesterol and its effects on heart health.)

Power of the mind to support your diet

If you continually tell yourself you *must* lose weight you will find it very difficult to do so without frequent lapses and emotional distress. Replace the word *must* as follows:

'It would be *preferable* for me to lose weight, and I'm giving it my best shot. Each day is a new beginning, and if I go off track, I can start again.'

If you find yourself eating a 'forbidden' food and saying things like 'I'm useless, I can't stick to the diet, so I might as well eat the rest', instead think 'I'm going to eat this chocolate and enjoy every bit of it'. In this way, you give yourself permission to enjoy your food, thereby feeling sufficiently comforted and staving off the desire to eat more.

I have extensively used imagery linked to relaxation either to encourage sensations of feeling full or to stimulate appetite for those who are either under-eating or rushing their food. If you cannot see in images, use your sense of smell and taste instead. Now think of the food you are going to have for lunch, read the following, and then close your eyes and try it:

Make yourself as comfortable as you can, allowing your hands to rest gently on your lap. If you can, close your eyes, take a deep comfortable breath and, as you breathe in, feel this wonderful oxygen pass down through your body.

As you breathe out, feel it pushing any tension or staleness out and away. Repeat this four times, and each time you will feel your body becoming more and more relaxed.

Feel your calves, knees and thighs soften, your tummy, back, shoulders, elbows, wrists and hands sink down.

Allow your head to rest gently on your shoulders, your lips to part slightly and the tongue to nestle in the lower part of the jaw.

Comfortable breathing now, not deep, picture your desired food, relish the smell it emits, stimulating your appetite. As you take a mouthful, see yourself enjoying its wonderful taste, passing gently down as you swallow, providing renewed energy and comfort.

Enjoy every mouthful, feel yourself becoming more and more comforted, relaxed, energized.

In your mind, say to yourself, ‘I have allowed this wonderful food to enter my body, to comfort me, to restore my energy. I feel good, I feel content, I feel full.’

12

Safe exercise

Heart conditions mostly strike people in their fifties or sixties, meaning that many of you reading this book will have been born between the 1940s and 1960s – eras when exercise was part of everyday lives, and sedentary lifestyles were relatively unheard of. I remember children's television being 3.30 p.m. to 5.30 p.m. each day and Saturday mornings. If you wanted to have recreation apart from these times, you played active games, outside. Was it like this for you? If so, you have a wonderful bank of memories of excitement, fun, freedom, stamina, companionship and, most importantly, feeling healthy. Belief was the key to exercise in your youth: belief that you could score that goal, could win that race, could enjoy exercise, taking risks and enjoying the consequences.

Rest assured I'm certainly not about to encourage you to take risks – quite the contrary – but I will demonstrate ways you can regain mental belief in your abilities to perform, at a pace and to a level that suit your needs, enhance the way you feel, and ultimately improve your health and well-being.

Many of you will already be sold on the importance of exercise; others may feel that they are too old, too ill, or just incapable of maintaining a programme of exercise that can keep them well during this 'secondary preventative' stage of recovery. I believe that unless it has been medically recommended that you do not exercise at all (rare in my experience), anyone can.

Yet two-thirds of men and three-quarters of women are not active enough, with 37 per cent of coronary heart disease deaths directly related to insufficient physical activity (BHF, 2005).

Many people I know, and most of those who took part in my questionnaire, believed that their inactive lifestyles contributed to their illness. As Marjorie explained, 'I never really did much exercise and I was always feeling tired, so I suppose I would judge myself to have been 4/10 fit. After my diagnosis, I started exercise classes and walking and now I feel 9/10 fit.'

Benefits of exercise

Exercise increases the efficiency of the heart by improving its blood supply, promotes circulation, lowers blood pressure and stores energy to combat fatigue. Regular exercise not only cuts the risk of premature death by a third, but halves the risk of a heart attack because the heart – like any other muscle when it receives regular exercise – grows stronger, the capacity of the lungs increases, and the heart pumps more blood with each beat.

Some of you may find this statement difficult to believe if you have been particularly active throughout your life and yet still developed a heart condition. Usually there are clear indications that this particular person has been either overly active or competitive, saw exercise as a 'must do it' or tended to have a yo-yo programme (lots at one time and then none). Usually too there has been clear evidence of stress or a previously unknown genetic condition.

Current health recommendations are that adults should take at least 30 minutes of moderate exercise on five or more days a week. Moderate physical activity is defined as causing an increase in breathing and higher heart rate, so that the pulse can be felt in the body alongside a feeling of increased warmth.

What exercise should you choose during your recovery?

Initially there are two programmes of exercise: one is a hospital-based rehabilitation programme, and the other is community-based rehab, exercise classes or personalized gym, walking or sports programmes.

Hospital-based programmes

These vary, but usually run for 6 to 12 weeks and can begin within a few weeks for those who have had a heart attack, or after three months for those who have had surgery. The main benefits of hospital courses include medical guidance, facilities, help at hand if needed, and the chance to be with others with a similar condition. Some rehab courses also offer the opportunity to learn about alternative therapies, as well as healthy heartcare.

Community-based programmes

Moving out into the community may be confusing or scary. Again, however, you have the opportunity to meet others with similar or differing experiences, and to feel 'normal' again.

Both sets of classes should teach you about breathing techniques, how to exercise correctly and safely at a pace that's right for you, and ultimately help you regain your confidence in a fun, non-competitive atmosphere where you have the opportunity to voice your experiences and discuss how your condition specifically affects you at this time.

In many cases, those who have joined such rehabilitation courses have been able to return to full-time work. It really depends on your age and the severity of your condition.

Make exercise part of your everyday life

Incorporating exercise into your daily routine is ideal. Walk where possible on your own or with others; use the stairs instead of the lift; take a break in the fresh air with a cool drink or a refreshing cup of tea; and when sitting use circulatory and relaxation techniques.

Additionally, try to incorporate exercise programmes into your lifestyle at least twice a week – join an exercise class on your own or with your partner, or take up another activity such as bowling or walking. Try to keep it up for at least an hour, but no more than two. Use background music to avoid boredom and to stimulate your ability to exercise for longer. Research has shown that listening to music while jogging keeps the mind alert, stimulating the release of the chemical called dopamine and of the 'feel-good' chemicals called endorphins.

Going to the gym

Many gyms, sports centres and health clubs also provide exercise tutors trained to work with people with a heart condition.

Many older people do not like the sole use of gym equipment. For some, it encourages them to overdo it, while most of those I have watched and spoken to do not understand the importance of breathing throughout an exercise – in fact, this is the main problem. They tend to concentrate so hard on getting the number of repetitions or time completed right that they forget to breathe and instant fatigue sets in.

If you are going to the gym, make sure you practise the breathing technique (see page 46) and use it throughout the exercises. For example, breathe normally, and on every fourth repetition take a deeper breath and exhale slowly and deeply. Crucially, remember if you feel dizzy you are either working too fast, you are holding your breath, or you have not breathed out sufficiently.

Do make sure when first using gym equipment that you have an introductory session with a qualified trainer who should design a specific training programme for you (ask for it in writing). You should be taught to break each technique down into understandable and attainable portions. Do check out that your tutor is *properly qualified*. If you have any concerns, you can take the name of their professional body and contact them.

If you intend to eat at the gym, check out whether it has healthy foods and supplies drinking water or at least sells bottles of it. Better still, make your own sandwich to take with you and leave a bottle of water overnight in the fridge.

For those who have suffered 'heart failure', where conventional exercise routines are too strenuous, contact the BHF for information on a tai chi project which provides a gentle but sustained exercise regime. (See Useful addresses.) Or try my simple warm-up exercise routine on page 108.

I actually enjoy both exercising with others and using gym equipment. You too can do this if you keep to the following simple rules to ensure safety and enjoyment.

Exercise safely

- **ALWAYS check with your heart consultant or GP before you join an exercise class or gym**. In most cases it is safe to do so from between six weeks to three months, depending on your individual circumstances. However, anyone can carry out the simple, circulatory exercises as soon as they come home from hospital.
- **ALWAYS inform your tutor of your condition**. Say how long it has been since you last exercised and any particular physical difficulties that you have.
- **ALWAYS warm up and cool down**. Warming up is the most important aspect of safety in any sport as it prepares the joints for work, improves the circulatory system by raising body tempera-

ture and blood flow to the working muscles, and prepares nerve and muscle response patterns, thus preventing muscle soreness and injury. Consult a trained tutor or see my warm-up programme in Chapter 13. Always cool down after exercise by walking for between five and ten minutes, which allows the heart and circulation to naturally slow down.

- **ALWAYS wear appropriate clothing and footwear**. Buy a good pair of trainers with non-slip soles, providing comfort and support – especially around the ankles. Keep clothing loose – preferably several layers with cotton next to the skin, so that you can strip off a layer if you get hot. Jogging bottoms or shorts should have an elasticated waistband, otherwise your movement capacity will be restricted. Don't wear jewellery: it can be a real hazard.
- **ALWAYS pace yourself**. Begin slowly, increase pace during the middle sections, and slow down towards the end of your exercise programme. Many people believe that as they have most energy at the beginning of their exercise or sport, that is when they should put most energy in, but your body will work more efficiently if it is allowed to slowly increase the pace. Do not over-exert yourself; you will tire easily and may injure yourself. The object is to feel revitalized, not drained. In the same vein, do not compete with others. This does not mean that team games or competitive situations are wrong, merely that understanding your own capabilities is imperative before you enter such a situation.
- **ALWAYS incorporate stretching into any exercise routine**. Stretching is essential to prepare muscles to contract and expand. In my classes I ensure that deep breathing with a stretch is used between more strenuous exercises to provide a calming break, develop posture, and enable the muscles to develop natural contraction and expansion motions.
- **LISTEN to your body**. If you are extremely breathless or take a long time to recover after exercise, you are working too hard. Always take breaks when you feel tired or particularly uncomfortable.
- **CHOOSE an activity that you enjoy**. You're much more likely to stick with it.
- **CHOOSE your best time of day to exercise**, but don't overdo it (see 'pace yourself', above).
- **NEVER hold your breath in order to work faster**. I have seen so many people holding their breath while exercising because they

believed they could work faster, for longer, or they didn't realize they were doing it. Yet this is counter-productive, as it stops the heart performing at its peak. In the past, going for the 'burn' (not achievable unless you held your breath), was considered to be the ultimate evidence of having worked hard. In fact, it is evidence of having worked *too* hard, causing a build-up of lactic acid, which basically burns the muscle. If you have previously held this belief about the 'burn', forget it. When completing an exercise where you are bent over, ensure that you rise slowly, and deep breathe as you do so because getting up quickly requires increased blood flow and is often the reason for dizziness.

- **NEVER work through pain** or exercise a body part that is inflamed, tender or emits intense heat (see box below).

Pain

- Pain is a **warning** to stop what you are doing as it is likely to cause an injury.
- Listen to your body, act upon its messages, reduce the workload and deep breathe. A good exercise session should make you feel more energised, not exhausted or unable to walk.
- Recognize that most discomfort, or even pain, is rarely experienced immediately after exercise. It is usually felt a few days later and is called 'delayed onset muscle soreness'. Some people believe 'only if we feel sore the next day do we know that we have worked hard'. This is not true: in fact it is the opposite; if you feel good but not sore, then you know that the level of the activity was right for you, and then, and only then, should you work to develop it. If, however, you do experience some soreness, which is not unusual at first if you haven't exercised for some time or you are at the early stages of your recovery, a warm shower or a soak in the bath is very helpful as it relaxes muscles and soothes soreness.

Make sure you drink enough fluid

Many people don't drink enough while exercising. Do not undertake strenuous exercise without drinking enough fluid as it can lead to feeling nauseous and light-headed, and eventually will result in fatigue or even heat stroke. Drink at least half a litre of water half an hour before you begin to exercise because on average we lose 1 litre of fluid for every hour we exercise. Listen to your body; the more you sweat, the more fluid you lose and will need to replace.

Sip frequently when taking a break or moving from one piece of apparatus to another. Check the colour of your urine. If it is pale and plentiful, you are well hydrated, but if it's dark and in short supply, start drinking.

DON'T'S

- Do not exercise if you feel unwell. However, if you are suffering from depression, exercise will lift your spirits.
- Scar tissue can sometimes be painful and may cause some discomfort while exercising. Be cautious, but once the scar tissue has stretched and healed, any pain will cease.
- Do not try to keep up with others if you are overweight because during weight-bearing activities your body weight increases the load on muscles, tendons, ligament and joint structures. Be realistic and adapt the regime to the level and pace that is right for you. As you become stronger and lose weight, you will be able to increase the regime.
- Do not continue to exercise if you feel nauseous, dizzy or in pain. Stop.
- Do not eat a heavy meal shortly before you exercise. Allow at least two hours to digest; half an hour for a snack. When we eat, the heart pumps blood to the stomach in order to help it digest food. If we then exercise before the body has had time to do its job, the heart has to divert the blood from the stomach to the other areas of the body, which may cause you to feel sick or have indigestion. It is also best not to eat while exercising for the same reasons.
- Initially during your recovery, avoid exercising when it is very cold or hot or if you are living or holidaying at high altitudes.
- Do not over-exercise.
- Do not drink alcohol before or immediately after exercise as it can cause dehydration and slow down recovery from any injury.
- Do not chew gum or any food while exercising.
- I'm sure I'm preaching to the converted, but just in case you have used them in the past, do not use anabolic steroids (known as Anadrolone) to increase muscle strength and size and decrease

body fat. While it is true that they are initially effective at developing muscle tissue, increasing strength and improving the body's capacity to train and compete by reducing fatigue and recovery time, persistent use will cause damage to the major organs, particularly the liver and the heart, which grows when the drug is taken.
- Know when to say 'no more'; understand your limitations and accept you have good and bad days.

Exercises to avoid

I suggest you *avoid completely* the following exercises, which in certain individuals – and definitely as we get older – can cause injury:

- Toe touches, which are performed as ballistic (bouncy-jerky) stretches, forcing the knees to over-extend, placing tremendous pressure on the lower back. If knees are slightly bent – with a static stretch – this is an acceptable exercise but beware of the hazard.
- Straight leg sit-ups, which mainly use the hip flexors and can place undue strain on the lower spine as the back hyper-extends.
- Raising both legs at the same time, which can cause strain on the spine.
- Deep knee bends, as forceful stretching of the ligaments of the knee takes away its protection, leaving it open to injury.
- Sit-ups with your hands clasped behind your head, creating tension and pressure on the upper spinal column.
- Fast head and neck movements, complete head circling or tipping the head right back.
- Leaning backwards; ensure that any forwards or sideways bending or rotation of the spine is practised with bent knees.
- Twisting movements with a flat back, as it strains the lower back; extended arms add to the danger.

Dealing with injury as a result of exercise

There are many sports injuries clinics and over-the-counter treatments, but I would urge you to seek medical assistance before you self-treat. The only exception to this advice is to use *cold* water, either by immersing the injured part in it or by placing a cold compress on an area that hurts.

Back pain can also be relieved with both hot and cold treatments and with a simple exercise practised while lying on the floor or bed. The firmer the surface the better. I practise this one in the bath after I have been gardening:

1 Lie down, back flat on the floor, raise your knees up over your tummy as much as you can.
2 When your back feels flat down, lower your feet on to the ground but keep your knees bent.
3 Take a deep breath in, pushing the small of your back into the floor. Your pelvis will tilt (i.e. your bottom will rise slightly) as you breathe out; let it relax back.

Repeat this ten times.

Now that safety and preparation have been considered, we're ready to take some action, so read on! The next chapter explains how to start exercising.

13
Let's get moving

Look at the following classifications relating to stages of recovery and decide which one is you at this time:

Stage 1: for those who are still recovering from a recent illness or who have not exercised for some time.

Stage 2: for those who are in the early stages of recovery, but were fairly fit before they became ill, or whose illness has not left them with major debilitating effects. Some people are ready for this stage within a few weeks; others need longer, e.g. 3 months.

Stage 3: my students have usually been with me between 6 and 12 months when they reach this stage.

Week 1 to week 6 after discharge (applicable to all stages of recovery)

As you are in the early stages of recovery, the thought of exercising is probably the last thing on your mind, but there are simple circulatory and breathing exercises that will assist your recovery.

Ankle flexes

Sit comfortably in a chair with legs either on the floor or supported by a stool. Lift one foot up and support your upper leg with your hands. Circle the ankles 6 times one way and then six the other. Now bring the toes towards you (you will feel the calf muscle pull) and point away from you; repeat 4 times. Repeat the whole exercise with the other ankle. Do this every now and again whenever you are sitting down. It improves circulation and helps to disperse fluid from around the ankles. If you have scar tissue on your leg and it pulls when you try this, cut the number of repetitions to 4 for each ankle until the tissue has healed. Make this a lifetime exercise.

Try not to sit with your *ankles crossed* as you are preventing the blood circulating properly by exerting pressure (weight) from one foot on to the other. Every time you become aware they are crossed, uncross them and do the ankle circling.

Exercises to improve circulation

Many people complain of coldness, stiffness or pain in the fingers, hands and arms.

Using your thumb as the resting point, touch one finger at a time against it; repeat at least 4 times for each finger, both hands at the same time. Now open and close the fingers 10 times. Lastly, make one hand into a fist and rub the fist against the palm of the other hand. When it feels warm, place that heated fist on the outside part of the fingers on the other hand.

If your arms feel stiff, circle your wrists 4 times one way and 4 times the other, then stretch them out in front of you (shoulder height), hold for 4 seconds and lower; repeat 4 times.

Keeping the feet moving as you practise the upper body standing exercises, and walking around between exercise routines helps to improve blood circulation by preventing the blood from settling in the legs which causes the calves to ache (known as 'pooling').

Cramp

While cramp is painful, it is merely the muscle going into spasm. You need to stretch out the muscle to release the spasm. Either:

- Do it yourself: grab your toes and force them towards you, or stand up, put one foot in front of the other so that the leg with the cramp is stretched out behind and the foot is pressed into the (preferably cold) floor.

Or:

- Get your partner to hold your foot and press your toes towards you (this stretches out the calf where cramps are usually felt) while at the same time rubbing the calf muscle gently to stimulate and restore the blood flow.

Some people find they can prevent cramps by having a warm shower first thing in the morning, or practising the ankle flexing exercise before they get in or out of bed.

Pelvic squeeze

Leaking from our passages can be distressing, but is common, and can be reduced in severity by strengthening the muscles around this area. Practise this simple exercise ten times while sitting, repeated at least five times a day, and let it become a lifetime exercise.

Pull in your muscles from your front to your back passage, feel them pull up inside you, breathe while you hold them, and then release. This can be repeated anywhere, at any time of the day.

There are different visual aids that may help you:

1 Think of a banana and imagine peeling it as you pull the muscles up inside you.
2 Imagine you are about to meet an important person and you want to pass wind; what do you do!
3 Imagine you are in a lift; each time you reach a different floor, pull the muscles in a little more. Say to yourself, 'Pull in 1st floor, pull in 2nd floor, pull in 3rd floor, release'.

One way of checking if you are getting better is to test yourself as you pass water. If you can stop the flow in mid-stream you will feel your muscles pull up. **Warning**: do not repeat this more than once a month, as you could cause an infection.

Other exercise regimes

The following exercise regimes can be undertaken in two stages.

The first part, done *sitting*, can be used on its own during the early stages of recovery to build muscle strength and flexibility.

The second part, done *standing*, can be introduced one to three months into your recovery, depending on your limitations, and can become an effective warm-up routine that you can use at any time to prepare for more strenuous exercise.

The sitting exercises

Simple shoulder, ankle and knee exercises linked to breathing will help to reduce stiffness from sitting and aid any chest wound to stretch and heal.

Sit on the edge of the seat and slowly 'walk' your bottom backwards until it touches the back of the chair. Allow your back to unfold and press firmly against the back of the chair.

Try to remember to breathe before you attempt each exercise. If you feel dizzy, you are not breathing out sufficiently; next time, make the out breath longer.

If you are at **stage 1**, practise these sitting exercises every other day for the first month, and then every day for the next two months. If you are at **stage 2**, practise these sitting exercises every day. If you are at **stage 3**, you can use these exercises permanently, *plus* the standing exercises, as an adequate warm-up and circulation programme for all other exercise regimes.

If you can, get someone to read the instructions out to you.

Neck rotation (slow movements)

1 Sitting upright with your head in a central alignment, take a breath in. As you breathe out, lower your chin to chest. As you breathe in again, return your head to the centre position. As you breathe out, raise your eyes to the ceiling. As you breathe in, return to centre. Repeat 4 times.
2 Starting at the central position, take a deep breath in. As you breathe out, turn your head to one side as far as you comfortably can. As you breathe in, return to the centre position. As you breathe out, turn your head to the other side. As you breathe in, return to the centre. Repeat 4 times.
3 Starting at a central position, imagine you have a mayoral chain of office lying on your chest and you want to check that everything is still there. Take a deep breath in, then lower your head until you can see your left shoulder; then slowly, as you breathe out, allow your head to move down across your chest and up towards your other shoulder. Pause, then take a deep breath in, lower and, as you breathe out, return across the chest to the other shoulder. Repeat 4 times.

Shoulder circles As you take a deep breath in, lift one shoulder up towards your ear; as you breathe out, circle backwards and downwards, then repeat using alternate shoulders 4 times each. Then repeat the same breathing pattern as above, but move both shoulders at the same time. Repeat 4 times.

Shoulder stretches

1 Either clasping your hands together or placing one hand flatly in the palm of the other, take a breath in and stretch your arms out in front of you (arms stay at shoulder height), then breathe out holding the arms outstretched.

2 Continue to breathe in and out while the stretch is held for 8 seconds and lower arms to your sides.
3 If you feel able, breathe in and tilt your body to one side until you feel the stretch down your other side; breathe out while keeping the stretched position.
4 Continue to breathe in and out while the stretch is held for 8 seconds. Repeat for the other side and then sit up.

Other exercises while sitting Continue to do the circulation exercises of the feet and ankles.

Also, lift your knees up and down 10 times for each leg. Then repeat, but as each leg is lifted up, stretch it out in front of you. The action therefore is bend up, stretch out, bend back and lower.

The standing exercises

After looking at sitting, we now need to consider movement. The most important element is walking, which during the first few weeks of recovery may naturally cause you either discomfort or concern. Those in **stage 1** and **stage 2** need to practise the following every day for the next month:

- Ensure that every hour, or at least every two hours, you get up from your chair and *walk up and downstairs once*, making sure that you maintain good posture. Hold on to the banister, but stay tall and take as many breaths as you like. It is the same principle coming down, but ensure that your foot is securely on the step before you hold your body upright.
- If you have a garden, every two hours *walk outside* and slowly amble around looking at the plants, smell their wonderful aromas, listen to the sounds of the birds and generally enjoy the scene. If it is a small garden, walk around it at least 4 times; if it is large, do it twice; if it is enormous, walk with someone else and do it just once.
- Being outside and digging up the odd weed is very rewarding, but when you bend down, do not lean over with your legs straight. Put one foot in front of the other (balance) and bend at the knees.
- Housework is good as it keeps you moving, but keep it light; for example, before or after washing up, hold on to the sink, then raise first one heel and then the other one (like walking, but with the toes staying static on the floor). Repeat 10 times, then repeat again with both heels off the ground and lower; repeat 10 times –

this strengthens the calf muscles. Turn sideways, still holding on with one hand, and swing your outside leg up in front of you 4 times, to the side of the body 4 times, swinging back 4 times; keep your body upright at all times (posture). Turn around and repeat on the other leg.

Basic standing exercise warm-up programme This is suitable for those in **stages 1**, **2**, and **3**. If you are at **stage 1**, start these exercises after one month.

The following is a safe warm-up routine that you can easily practise at home, boosting circulation, flexibility, strength and breathing capacity and, when used with the relaxation section (see Chapter 14), it will add to your well-being. It can also be used with the exercise bike and walking programmes. Remember to always come back to the standing tall position after each exercise.

If practising these exercises indoors, ensure you have enough space to reach out in all directions.

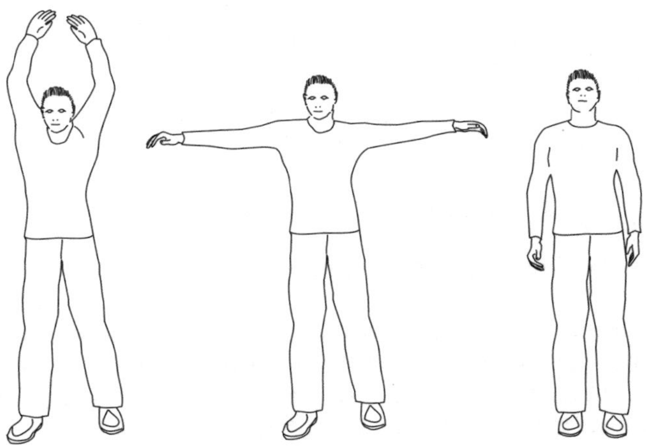

Figure 2 Arm swings

- Arm swings (see Figure 2)

Breathe in and swing your arms out to the sides and up as far as you can; breathe out as you lower them. Repeat 4 times.

If you cannot take a deep breath because of an operation scar or poor lung capacity, only reach up to a point that is comfortable. If you feel cold, practise the circulation exercises (see page 107).

- Shoulder circles

As you take a deep breath in, lift one shoulder up towards your ear; as you breathe out, circle backwards and downwards. Repeat using alternate shoulders, 4 times each.

Then repeat the same breathing pattern, but move both shoulders at the same time. Repeat 4 times.

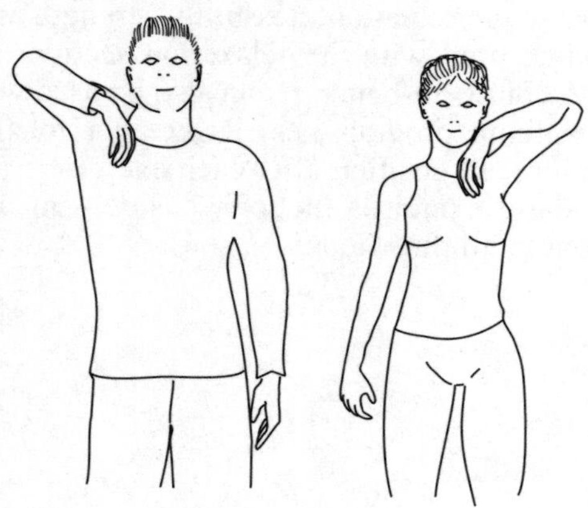

Figure 3 Elbow shoulder circles

- Elbow shoulder circles (see Figure 3)

As you take a deep breath in, bend your arm at the elbow and lift it up; as you breathe out, circle it backwards and down. Repeat with alternate shoulders 4 times. Use the same breathing pattern, but move both elbows at the same time. Repeat 4 times.

- Full arm swing (see Figure 4)

Take a breath in and swing one arm upwards; as you breathe out, lower it backwards (backstroke swimming action) and down. Repeat with alternate sides 4 times. Use the same breathing pattern, but swing both arms at the same time. If you have stiffness or it hurts your scar, start with small swings to the side; if you do not have a problem, try to get your arms as close to your ears as you can.

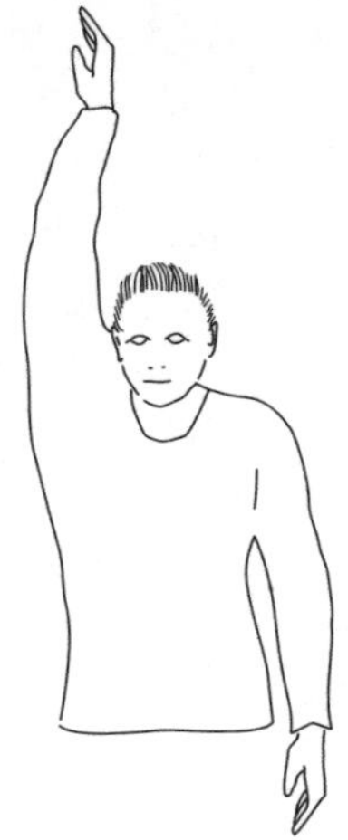

Figure 4 Full arm swing

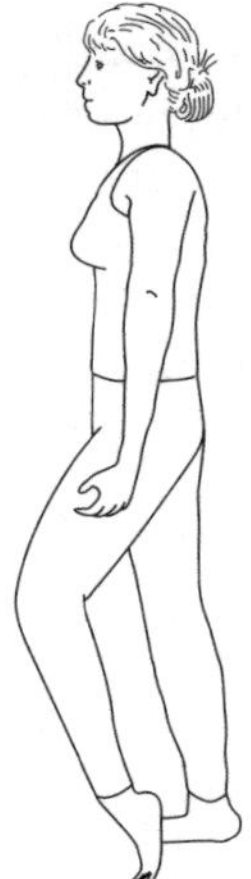

Figure 5a Ankle flexing

- Ankle flexing (see Figure 5a)

Have your feet flat on the floor, then raise and lower heels; keep toes on floor, slight knee bend, paying attention to your posture. Repeat 20 times. Do not rock back on your heels.

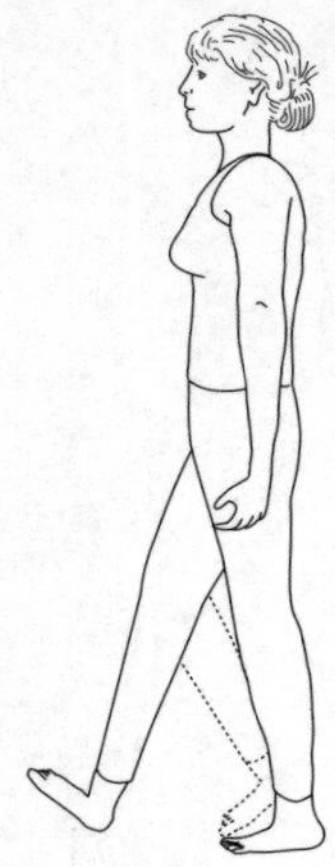

Figure 5b Ankle stretch

- Ankle stretch (see Figure 5b)

Stand tall. Reach out with one foot and place the heel down in front of your body, now back, touching floor with toes. Action is heel, toe, heel, toe. Repeat 20 times. Then repeat with the other foot.

You can develop the above into *ankle/calf stretch*. Heel touch in front of body, toe touch across other leg, heel touch in front of body, feet together. Repeat 10 times with each foot.

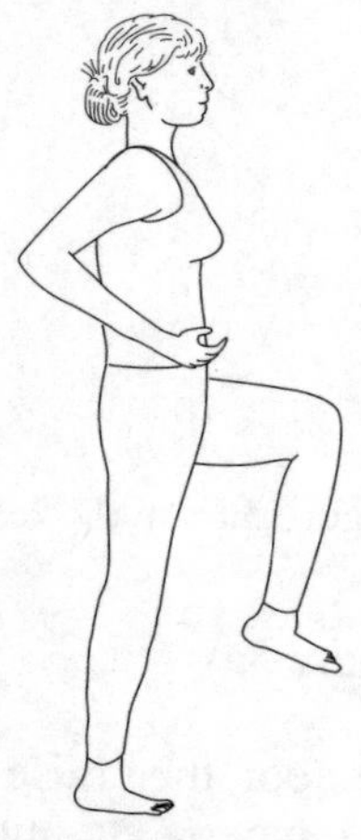

Figure 6 Knee lifts

- Knee lifts (see Figure 6)

Lift knees, one at a time, aiming to raise them to waist height. Keep body upright. Just lift as far as you can; do not force the lift if it hurts.

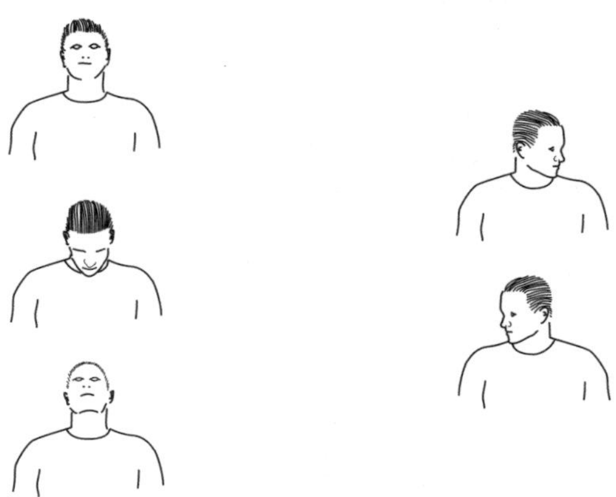

Figure 7 Neck rotation

- Neck rotation (slow movements) (see Figure 7)

With head in central alignment, take a breath in; as you breathe out, lower your chin on to your chest; as you breathe in again, return your head to the centre position; as you breathe out, raise your eyes to the ceiling; as you breathe in, return head to the centre. Repeat everything 4 times.

Starting at the central position, take a deep breath in; as you breathe out, turn your head to one side as far as you comfortably can; as you breathe in, return to the centre position; as you breathe out, turn your head to the other side; as you breathe in, return to centre. Repeat 4 times.

Starting at the central position, imagine you have a mayoral chain of office lying on your chest and you want to check everything is still there. Take a deep breath in, then lower your head until you can see your left shoulder; then slowly, as you breathe out, allow your head to move down across your chest and up towards your other shoulder.

Pause, take a deep breath in, lower your head, and as you breathe out return your head across your chest to the other shoulder. Repeat 4 times.

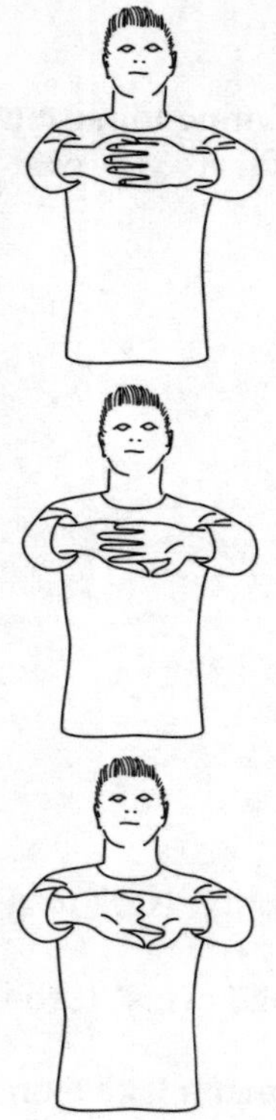

Figure 8 Further arm/shoulder exercises

- Arms/shoulders (see Figure 8)

Step 1 – if you have difficulty intertwining your fingers, place one hand flat inside the other, take a breath, and stretch your arms out in front of you (shoulder height); breathe out and hold the stretch for 8 seconds (do not hold your breath).

Step 2 – now turn your hands so that the palms face outwards as you stretch; include the breathing as for step 1 and hold the stretch for 8 seconds.

Step 3 – if you do not have a shoulder problem, intertwine your fingers, and as you breathe in, stretch your arms above your head; breathe out and hold the stretch for 8 seconds (breathe normally). Only do what is comfortable for you.

• Shoulder/upper arm stretch (see Figure 9)

Extend your arm out in front of you (shoulder height). Place your other hand on the elbow of the outstretched arm and gently pull across the body (keep arm straight). Hold for 8 seconds. Repeat on the other side.

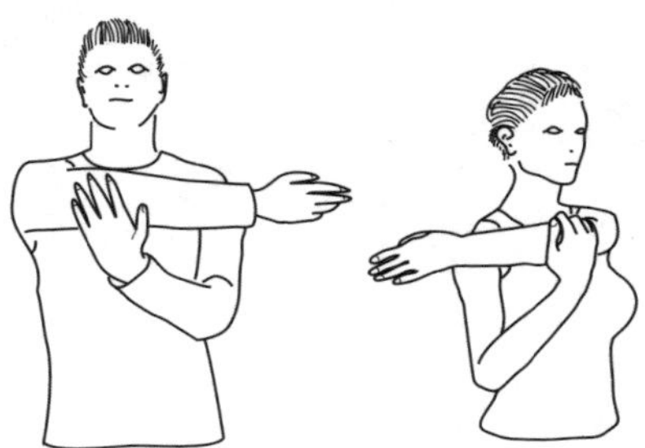

Figure 9 Shoulder/upper arm stretch

• Side extension (see Figure 10)

Stand upright, feet slightly turned out, and slightly bent at the knees.

Reach down one side and feel the stretch on the other. Hold the stretch for 8 seconds.

Repeat for the other side. Reach only to the point of feeling the stretch; do not over-reach.

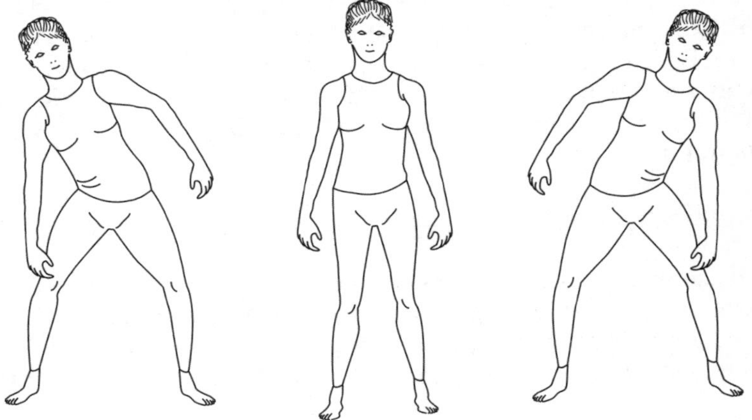

Figure 10 Side extension

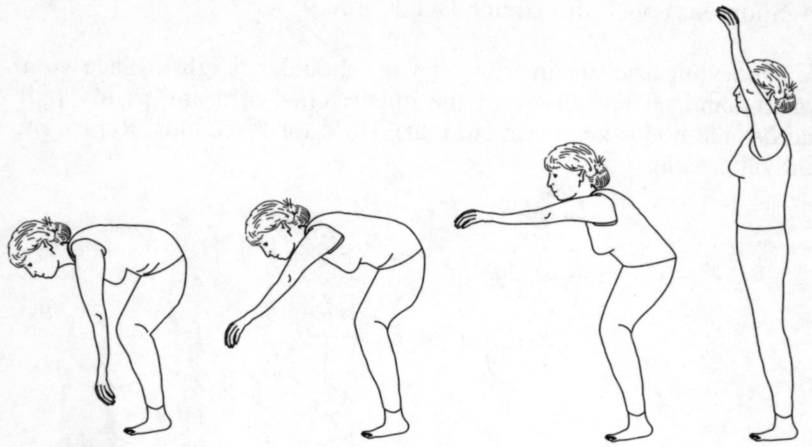

Figure 11 Back flexia

• Back flexia (see Figure 11)

Stand tall, arms above your head. Take a breath in and, as you breathe out, allow your arms to swing down towards your toes, at the same time bending at the knees. Repeat 4 times.

This is an excellent movement to stretch and relax the lower back before any strenuous exercise, or even just before gardening. However, **never** complete this action with straight legs. Note the different images; one is for those who have stiff backs or have not exercised for a while, the other is for those who have flexibility. Start with the first and slowly develop until you can reach the toes. If at the initial stage of recovery you feel dizzy when you try this, **do not** do it.

• Calf stretch (see Figure 12a)

Feet together, take one comfortable stride forward with one leg. Bend the knee on that leg, ensuring it is directly over the ankle. The back leg will be straight, foot facing forwards, and you will feel a stretch in the calf muscle. Hold for 8 seconds. Repeat with other leg.

• Achilles stretch (see Figure 12b)

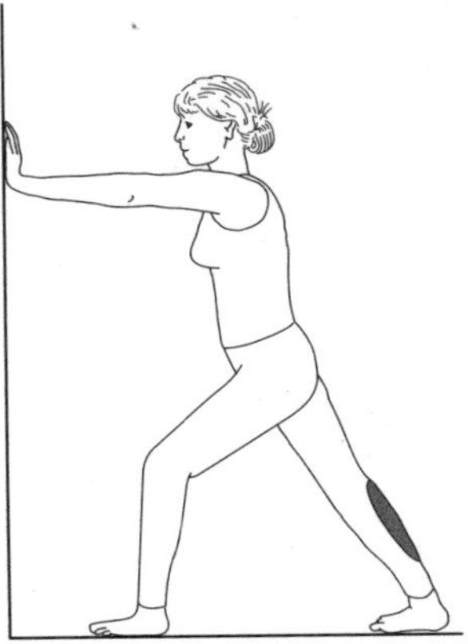

Figure 12a Calf stretch

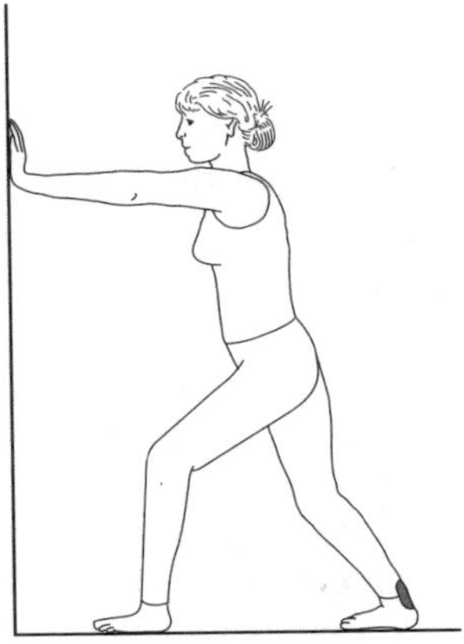

Figure 12b Achilles stretch

This is the same position, but now bend the back knee until you feel a stretch around the ankle. Hold for 8 seconds. Repeat with other leg. *Note*: if you feel unbalanced, ensure that you have a wider stance or place both hands against a wall.

It is inadvisable to practise the following exercises at home unless you have a wall that is free of furniture or you are able to hold on to a chair that can take your weight:

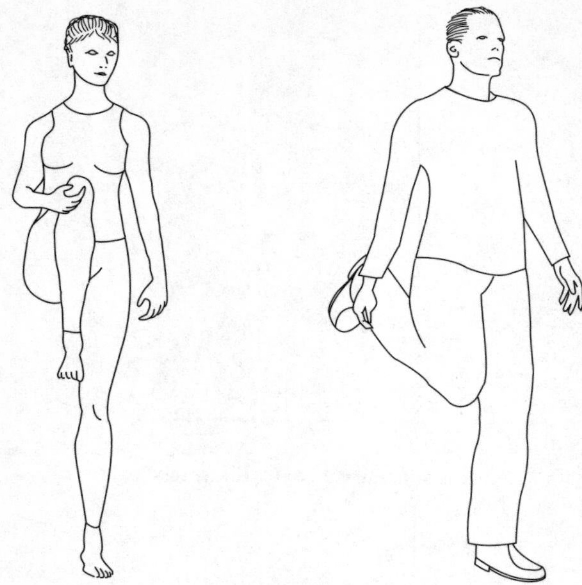

Figure 13 Hamstring/quads stretch

- Hamstring/quads stretch (see Figure 13)

Stand tall, lift the knee that is farthest from the wall as high as you can and, using your free hand, hold it into the chest for 8 seconds. Turn around and repeat with the other leg.

Hold on, and lift your heel up to your bottom; if you can, hold with your hand; if you cannot reach, do not force it – either hold on to clothing or just lift as high as you can. Hold for 8 seconds. Turn around and repeat for other leg.

- Leg swings/hip flexor

Stand tall, hold on, and swing your outside leg forwards 4 times, then sideways 4 times, and backwards 4 times.

At all times stay tall, do not lean forwards or backwards, and remember to breathe. Finally, walk around, either in your home or in the garden. If you have an exercise bike, cycle for five minutes.

Other exercise programmes to develop strength and improve health

Apart from exercises to do while sitting or standing, you can also benefit from other exercise programmes, including walking, swimming and using an exercise bike.

Walking

Here are some of the benefits of walking:

- After 10 to 15 minutes of walking, blood circulation in the brain has increased by 50 per cent, enabling you to think and concentrate better.
- The body burns approximately 100 calories per mile – the greater the incline, the more calories you burn.
- Visual surroundings enhance enjoyment, releasing serotonin, endorphins and anadamide (a substance found in the body when we are relaxed).
- Walking requires no equipment or expense.
- Latest research from the BHF reminds us that we need to take 10,000 steps a day to keep healthy – you can buy step monitors from most sports shops and chemists. Just be aware that everybody's step rhythms are different, so read the instructions carefully and set the monitor appropriately for your needs.

Walking programme

Walking is such a simple and natural activity, but many people with heart problems experience pain when walking, mostly because they set off with unrealistic expectations that do not take into account the length, duration or the inclines.

Always practise the warm-up routines before you go walking.

Let's take one step at a time.

1. Decide how long your walk will be, i.e. end of the road, round the block, 1 mile, 2 miles, 3 miles, etc. Or set a time limit, i.e. 10 minutes, 20 minutes, 30 minutes, etc. (remember that each time slot includes the return journey).
2. Initially choose a route that does not have many slopes and is enjoyable to look around at.
3. Start slowly, slower than your normal pace. The middle section of

your walk should be at your normal pace. Your heart is now ready to respond to the extra demands and there should be no pain. Slow down for the last section of your walk to give the body time to readjust to its 'impending rest' (cool down).

4 Aim to walk every day initially, and then at least 3 times a week for a set period of time or distance. Encourage a partner, friend or family member to join you.
5 Keep at the same distance/time until your body tells you it is becoming effortless.
6 Wear appropriate clothing depending on the weather; in particular, carry a scarf to cover your mouth (not your nose, unless extremely cold) if it is very windy and you suffer with chest pain.

Planning a progressive walking programme Listen to your body; it will tell you if you have overdone it, or indeed could do more. **Never** walk through pain; rest until the pain subsides and then continue (or return home) at a slower pace.

Initially you may only be able to walk as far as the garden gate. Deep breathe and walk slowly several times a day, increasing the distance until you can confidently walk to the end of the road and progress from there.

When you have progressed to a 3-mile (or longer) walk and that becomes easy, change your route so that you have to walk up an incline or two, or even steps.

When expanding your walks, I suggest that time limits are easier to adhere to than set distances. Try to ensure someone walks with you and if you are able to have a conversation on the return as well as the outward journey without becoming overly breathless, you can safely walk a little further or a little faster. In Chapter 16, I refer to six progressive walking programmes starting with Walk 1 (10 minutes), progressing as you grow stronger through to Walk 2 (20 minutes), Walk 3 (30 minutes), Walk 4 (40 minutes), Walk 5 (1 hour), and Walk 6 (1 hour but increasing your pace within the middle 10 minutes).

If you like to walk in groups, experience guided walks, or wish to organize such a group in your area, you can contact the Countryside Agency or the BHF which have information on existing groups and provide a booklet entitled *Practical Guidelines for Developing Walking for Health Schemes*.

Exercise bikes (for use at home)

Tips:

- Buy a good, sturdy, reliable bike.
- When you stand by the side of the bike, the seat should be the same level as your hip. Sit on it and if you find yourself having to lean over to one side to push the pedal down, the seat is too high. If you find your legs are not quite extended during the downward pedal action, the seat is too low. Adjust the seat so that the ball of the foot reaches the pedal with the leg straight in the lowered pedal position.
- Try to ensure that your arms are almost straight and your body is comfortable. If you find yourself leaning forwards so that there is body weight pushing on your arms, adjust the handlebars.
- Start off slowly at low or nil resistance.
- Some people prefer to cycle for a longer time, rather than with a firmer resistance.
- Don't use your exercise bike straight after a meal. Give your food time to digest (at least 30 minutes).
- It helps to keep the momentum going by watching television or listening to the radio while you cycle. Just be aware of the time and listen to your body.

Cycling programmes

1 *Beginning/basic* For those who are at stage 1 in their recovery, who have recently left hospital after an operation, have been unwell for some time, or have not exercised for months or years:

Stage 1 (weeks 1/2)
e.g. 5 minutes' cycling twice a day at **nil resistance**. (Nil resistance means that you are not using the brake system that makes pedalling harder.)
Steady pace, 5 minutes, morning and afternoon.
Continue every day for two weeks.

Stage 2 (weeks 3/4)
e.g. 10 minutes' cycling twice a day at **nil resistance**.
Steady pace, not fast, 10 minutes, morning and afternoon.
Continue every day for two weeks.

Stage 3 (weeks 5/6)
5 minutes' cycling twice a day at **slight resistance**.

(Slight resistance means you can feel a resistance to the pedalling action and you have to work harder.)
Steady pace, 5 minutes, morning and afternoon.
Continue every day for two weeks.

Stage 4 (weeks 7/8)
10 minutes' cycling twice a day at **slight resistance**.
Steady pace, 10 minutes, morning and afternoon.
Continue every day for two weeks.

After one month of the above programme some people will feel ready to move on to a more demanding programme; others need the full two months. If you do not feel ready to move on, continue as before for another month, repeating the **stage 4** programme.

2 *Development* This programme is suitable for those ready to extend their exercise routine to a greater degree of difficulty, or who are already attending an exercise class, but wish to exercise at home as well.

Stage 1 (weeks 1/2)
15 minutes' cycling twice a day or, if you work, 20 minutes' cycling once a day with **slight resistance**.
Set the resistance (brake) to your level of fitness, i.e. if your muscles feel very sore the day after exercise, then you have set the resistance too high, so lower it.
If after your time limit you feel that you could go on for much longer, try a higher resistance.
Continue every day for two weeks.

Stage 2 (weeks 3/4)
Either increased time or increased resistance (brake)
i.e. 20 minutes' cycling twice a day or, if you work, 25 minutes' cycling once a day with the **resistance set as for week 1**.
Or 15 minutes' cycling twice a day or, if you work, 15 minutes' cycling twice a day with **additional resistance**.

Stage 3 (weeks 5/6)
Either increased time or increased resistance (brake)
i.e. 25 minutes' cycling twice a day or, if you work, 30 minutes' cycling once a day with the **resistance set as for week 1**.
Or 20 minutes' cycling twice a day or, if you work, 30 minutes' cycling once a day – both with **additional resistance**.

Stage 4 (weeks 7/8)
Either increased time or increased time and resistance (brake)
i.e. 30 minutes' cycling twice a day or, if you work, 40 minutes' cycling once a day with the **resistance set as for week 1**.
Or 25 minutes' cycling twice a day or, if you work, 40 minutes' cycling once a day with **additional resistance**.

It is important to use your bike as an addition to walking, swimming or exercising, not as a replacement. As a general guideline once you are feeling fitter and healthier, twice a day for 30 minutes three times a week is an adequate programme to maintain your level of fitness.

Swimming

Swimming is an excellent overall exercise and a great family activity. It improves lung capacity, flexibility and stamina and helps with any weight loss; it is progressive and builds strength in a non-competitive atmosphere. But unless you are a competent swimmer, it is not advisable to begin swimming in the first few weeks of your recovery (and not in these early days if you have had surgery).

This section is written specifically for those of you who are either non-swimmers or who are nervous about 'how much to do'.

Progressive swimming programme

Stage 1 This is for non-swimmers and those who are recovering from an illness or operation. Always warm up by using a few of the guidelines in the warm-up programme (one for each part of the body). These can be done in the changing room (be careful if it is only a cubicle) or in the water (a wonderful way to tighten those loose muscles, reduce fat and give your body a nice firm shape).

- Always enter in the shallow end of the pool.
- Remember that the body needs time to prepare itself.
- Start by walking across the width of the pool (not too quickly) as if you were walking in the street – twice.
- If it feels comfortable, lower your body until your shoulders are just under the water and walk across the pool again.
- Hold on to the gully at the side of the pool, and raise and lower your body up to your shoulders 10 times (not too quickly).

- Go through the warm-up exercises for the legs, e.g. ankle flexes, leg raises, sideways, forwards.
- Hold on to the gully with your arms (back to the side of the pool) – be careful if your operation scar is still sore – and raise your legs in front of you, either doing a cycling action with your legs or gentle kicking. Do this 10 times.
- Turn on to your front, hold on to the side with one hand, place your other hand lower down against the wall (better support), arms outstretched, and allow your legs to raise up behind you and gently kick. Non-swimmers do not be afraid, you will not sink; all you have to do is lower the feet to stand up again. Repeat 10 times.
- Now aim to swim across the width of the pool doing the breaststroke action. (If this hurts your leg scar, you may find it easier to do the crawl leg action.) The breaststroke arm action is thought to be the least painful action for the chest scar.
  Or:
  Swim across with a floating action (on your back), lay back, arms by your side, and using your hands draw a figure eight and gently kick with your legs. Be careful, as in this position you cannot see the side of the pool. Non-swimmers – on your back, hold a float across your chest or behind your head and kick with your feet.
- Initially use the breaststroke action in preference to the crawl, as it is slower and is less worrying because the face is out of the water.
- If you cannot swim or your chest is sore, ask the pool attendant for a float (or buy your own).
- Initially rest after the completion of each width (do not worry if you need to stop during the width, this will improve in time). Take 5 deep breaths.
- Do not stay in the water once you have completed your swim.

Start by going swimming once a week and aim to complete 4 widths, gradually progressing to 10 widths once a week over the next ten weeks. There are many beginners swimming classes available, and a few classes specifically for those who have been unwell or are disabled. Contact your nearest community education centre for details.

Stage 2 After 10 weeks, if you are able to complete 10 widths without discomfort, you can progress to the following:

- Aim to complete 2 of the 10 widths continuously before you take a break and deep breathe 5 times.
- Add 1 width each week to your continuous swimming programme until you are able to complete 10 widths without the need for a break.

  Remember: consciously breathing throughout your swimming makes it easier and improves stamina.
- Once you can do 20 continuous widths, alter your stroke with each width, e.g. breaststroke, backstroke, front crawl, floating.

Stage 3 Warm up as before. Swimming lengths: always swim from the deep end to the shallow end. Should you feel unable to complete a length, you will then be able to walk the rest.

- After your warm-up, get out of the pool and walk to the deep end. Walk down the steps and immediately swim towards the shallow end, using any stroke. Breathe.
- Nervous swimmers should aim to keep about 3 feet from the edge of the pool; they will then be able to hold on if they need to rest.
- Repeat the above routine 5 times, progressing gradually over the weeks to 10 lengths. Always walk slowly from the shallow to the deep end.

When you are able to complete 10 lengths with ease, start swimming 2 lengths continuously before you have a rest. This time, start from the shallow end. Rest for at least a minute or two, take a few deep breaths, and begin again. The rest period depends on how far you wish to extend yourself.

Eventually you will find you are able to swim 10 lengths without a break. It is not important how quickly you complete the lengths, just as long as you do them.

This gradual progression takes time – for some people a couple of months, for others a year. Remember you are not competing with anyone; you are assisting your recovery by becoming fitter and healthier in both body and mind.

The aim is for you to improve circulation, lung capacity, stamina and strength in an enjoyable and relaxing manner. Therefore, it does not matter if you never progress beyond stage 1. Why not just repeat stage 1 twice a week instead of moving on to stages 2 or 3?

Gauging how well you are doing with any exercise programme is easily done by listening to your body, but some people like to have evidence. One way of achieving this is to keep a diary for six months, noting down at the end of each week what you have achieved, how you felt before and afterwards, and grading your level of fitness.

For example, Stephen's diary looked like the one in Table 13.1:

Table 13.1 Diary for keeping track of your exercise routines

Date	*Level of fitness (out of 10) to begin with*	*Exercise I have done (number of repetitions)*	*Date: end of the week*	*Level of fitness (out of 10)*	*How I feel now*
Week 1: 1 March 2000	3	Warm-up sitting exercises and walking in garden twice a week	7 March 2000	4	Still very tired and fed up, but it has eased a bit
Week 12: 6 June 2000	6	Warm-up sitting and standing exercises every other day and walking 3 miles a day	12 June 2000	7	So much better, not so tired, stayed up longer last night than I have been able to before, chest has eased, breathing has really helped. Walked on my own this week. Great

Power of imagery in exercise

Many sportspeople use visualization to help the subconscious to relax. So next time you are thinking of exercising, close your eyes, take a couple of deep breaths, and see yourself doing it. Open your eyes and start to actually do so.

Lastly, do think about the exercise or sport you want to try, in relation to your previous experience and your ability to cope with such a regime. While it is true that we can all learn sports skills, there are inhibitors that can take away enjoyment. Be aware of any physical limitations that you may have, listen to your body, and learn to adapt the exercises accordingly.

14

Relaxation techniques

Relaxation does not come easily to most of us, mainly because we are not practised in listening to our body's inner messages. Relaxation may even sometimes appear to have superficial health benefits, but in fact can be our strongest support. It helps counterbalance levels of unmanageable pressure that can lead to stress by acting as a safety valve for mind and body. With the help of relaxation, tension drops and is replaced by calmness, control, confidence, increased concentration, and more energy. It also clears the mind of everyday negative thoughts, improves relationships, and provides time to concentrate on well-being and health. Most importantly, relaxation has been shown to be effective in lowering blood pressure, and is therefore often linked to a reduction in coronary artery disease.

Relaxation is powerful in its own right, but when linked with other de-stressors its effect can be greatly enhanced. So don't just read this chapter in isolation – have a look at the stress-beating techniques in Chapter 4 too!

Understanding a tense body

Muscular tension is necessary for everyday living, but it can become dangerous when it is not used for work, is frequently repeated, and inhibits the body's natural desire to relax. Tension has a counterproductive effect on health as it keeps adrenaline at high levels in the blood, slowing down the repair of tissue and the renewal of cells. Such levels of tension-related adrenaline are found to be reduced during relaxation or sleep. When recovering from surgery, relaxation supports the healing of skin cuts and wounds, and tension retards healing.

Preparing to relax

With practice, relaxation is achievable in seconds through either passive or active states:

- *Passive.* This is when relaxation is controlled by an exterior force such as massage, reflexology or aromatherapy, which work by creating internal energy from an external force.
- *Active.* This is when you yourself activate the relaxed feelings, for example with yoga, deep breathing, meditation or visualization.

Relaxation can be practised anywhere at any time, but when it involves anything over five minutes it would benefit you to consider the following:

- Choose a quiet environment, but be aware that noise may suddenly occur; with practice, you will be able to ignore it.
- Some people prefer a darkened room, others prefer light.
- If you suffer with aches or pains you may find relaxation lying down difficult. Choose instead a comfortable chair or sit against a wall with a cushion that supports your neck, head and shoulders.
- If closing your eyes is difficult, start with your eyes closed and open them whenever you need to.
- If you are using a spoken relaxation tape, choose one whose voice tone and use of words suits you. Some tapes offering to take you on a 'guided journey' may stir up sad or difficult memories; if so, either change the image it creates or do not use the tape.
- Start with the shorter relaxation processes such as deep breathing before you experience the longer 10- to 20-minute relaxation.

Never get up quickly.

Relaxation scripts

I do find that a relaxation script is very effective, and you'll find two below – one to be used while sitting, and one while lying down (choose the more comfortable one for you). Bear in mind that looking at a written script has its limitations, so it is a good idea to record yourself reading the scripts, or ask someone you know to record the scripts in an even, calming voice, so that you can play them back (or see Useful Addresses if you want to contact me for a personalized tape).

Breathing-enhanced relaxation

Ensure you are in a warm, quiet room with the light off or dimmed. Prepare yourself.

Sitting in a chair

Sit upright with the small of your back against the back of the chair, hands on your lap or on the arms of the chair. Remove your glasses if you wear them and close your eyes – if you feel any sense of discomfort, you can open your eyes at any time.

Have your feet flat on the floor, slightly apart, with your ankles and heels directly under your knees.

If at any time during this relaxation you are disturbed and need to deal with a situation quickly, open your eyes, take a deep breath and rise slowly.

Breathe naturally and comfortably throughout the exercises.

Now, read or record the following yourself, or ask a friend to do so (dots mean slight pauses):

Feet: Take a breath and, as you breathe out, allow your feet to sink down…into the floor.
Calves: Take a breath and, as you breathe out, feel those calf muscles soften…allow any tension to just melt…away.
Thighs: Take a breath and, as you breathe out, allow your thighs to soften…and sink gently into the seat.
Buttocks/stomach: Take a breath and, as you breathe out, allow the buttocks to part…the stomach to relax and your back to rest gently…against the back of the chair.
Hands/arms: Take a breath and, as you breathe out, feel your shoulders…elbows…wrists…and your hands sink…down.
Neck/head: Allow the head to rest securely on your shoulders…your eyes to sit gently in their sockets…the teeth to nestle in your mouth…the lips to part slightly and your tongue to rest…in the lower part of the jaw.
Now breathe: Take 8 deep breaths, allowing that wonderful oxygen to enter into your body, relaxing you more…and more…and more…

Lying down

Make yourself comfortable on a bed, couch, carpet or relaxation mat. Keep your body straight, head in alignment, arms by your sides. Remove your glasses and close your eyes (if you feel any sense of discomfort, you can open your eyes at any time).

Have a cushion under your head/neck or small of the back if you suffer back pain.

Remember to breathe at your own pace; do not hold your breath. Again, the dots in the script mean slight pauses.

Feet: Take a deep breath and, as you breathe out, let your feet drop away from you. They may feel heavy…heavy…heavy…becoming lighter…lighter…and lighter…
Calves: Take a deep breath and, as you breathe out, feel your calf muscles soften…feel any tension just melt…away.
Knees and thighs: As you breathe in, turn your knees and your thighs out to the side. As you breathe out, allow them to sink down into the floor. Take another breath and, as you breathe out, let them sink down lower…and lower, feeling lighter…lighter…and lighter, warmer…warmer…and warmer…more…and more…relaxed.
Tummy: Take as many breaths as you like. Each time you breathe out, feel your tummy muscles soften…and sink down into the floor. Feel the whole area become more…and more…relaxed, any tension just ebb…away.

Just for a moment let's concentrate on that wonderful oxygen. Take a deep breath in, feel that wonderful oxygen pass down through the stomach, thighs, calves, ankles and your toes and, as you breathe out, feel any remaining tension or staleness just leave…the body. Repeat 4 times.

Shoulders: As you breathe in, raise your right shoulder up towards your ears. Breathe out and let your shoulder pull down and away from the neck…allow your arm to rest at your side, turn your palm up to the ceiling, feeling the shoulder drop down even more…repeat the same for the left shoulder.

Just for a moment let's concentrate on that wonderful oxygen. Take a deep breath in, feel that wonderful oxygen pass down through the neck, shoulders, elbows, wrists and your hands as you breathe out, and feel any remaining tension or staleness just leave the body. Repeat 4 times.

Head/face: Gentle natural breathing now, not deep. Move your eyebrows up and away from your eyes…as you do so, feel the skin around your eyes soften…your lashes barely touch your cheeks. Allow your forehead to soften and drift…back into your hairline. Let your worries just drift…away. Feel the skin around your face soften...your lips part slightly...the jaw drop down towards the chest and the tongue to nestle in the lower part of the jaw.

Take a deep breath in, feeling that wonderful oxygen passing down through the whole of your body and, as you breathe out, feel any remaining tension or staleness just leave...the body. Repeat 4 times.

Feel that wonderful oxygen going deep...deep...down into your nerve endings, relaxing you more...and more...and more... Enjoy and relax.

Coming out of relaxation

It is essential to come out of relaxation slowly:

- Wiggle your fingers and your toes.
- Rub your hands together until you feel the warmth in your palms.
- Place these palms gently over your eyes.
- Open your eyes, and feel the warmth from your palms.
- Remove your palms from your eyes and look around you.

If sitting:

- Lift your heels up and down gently.
- Stretch your fingers and release.
- Lift your shoulders up to your ears, circle backwards and downwards and relax. Stand up and have a good stretch, raising your arms above your head and then lowering them.
- Walk around.

If lying down:

- Take a breath and slowly bring your knees towards you and place your feet on the floor.
- Wait a moment.
- Take a breath and slowly roll over on to your side (one whole movement, shoulder, hips and knees at the same time).
- Wait a moment.
- Take a breath and slowly come up to a sitting position.
- Wait a moment.
- Take a breath and move on to your knees, then stand up (if necessary, ensure there is a stable object such as a chair to support you as you rise).

Imagery

Imagery, an invaluable tool, is even more effective if you are relaxed.

There are many ways to use imagery to enhance and deepen a relaxed state, but the one I use the most is an approach I call 'personal journey'. After practising the full relaxation, imagine a favourite scene or take yourself on a journey using your five senses, such as:

- Imagine seeing oxygen as small tiny bubbles, soft floating clouds or a warm soft breeze. Take a deep breath in, feel the warmth, feel refreshed and, as you breathe out, push any staleness out through your feet.
- In your mind, see yourself going on a journey to a favourite place or somewhere you have always wanted to go. Look around you, soak up the sights, smells, sounds and tastes, and allow them to enter your body. Feel yourself relax more and more. Enjoy yourself.
- Imagine you are on a bed of soft feathers that are completely taking your weight.
- Feel the soft, floating sensation of weightlessness.
- Think of an object, a piece of furniture, china, etc., then visualize and feel the texture of this object.
- Visualize a piece of gold, silver or crystal, and watch it change shape and colour as the sun shines on it, feeling the warmth of the rays as they are reflected on to you.
- See yourself drawing or painting a picture using any medium, then step back and admire it.
- Imagine baking a cake or cooking a meal, then lie back and wallow in the smell and taste.
- Imagine listening to your favourite piece of music; allow it to soothe and calm you (preferably instrumental music as voices tend to raise and lower awareness, creating tension).
- See your favourite flowers emerge from a bud to a full flower, feel the strength inside you as they grow stronger and stronger.

If you cannot see in images, recite a favourite poem or indeed create positive sentences about yourself and your ability to assist the healing process

Record the sound of birds singing or water running, or buy a relaxation tape that provides such comforts.

Other ways to relax

There are many ways to relax once you feel well enough – art, music, dance, and so on. Laughter is also a natural relaxant; it lights up the face, makes us look younger, provides rapid relief from tension, releases endorphins into the bloodstream, and opens doors of friendship.

French neurologist Henri Rubenstein, who has studied laughter extensively, concludes that one minute of laughter provides up to 45 minutes of relaxation. This is reinforced by UK researchers, who say that 30 minutes of laughter a day is a strong inhibitor of a second heart attack.

Do you have any old videos or films that make you laugh? If not, go out and buy some, or let others provide them for you as get-well gifts.

Just remember that laughter always makes the chest 'wobble' and may therefore initially pull on any scar tissue, but it won't do it any harm. The benefits are far greater than any problems – just use a cushion pressed gently against the chest as you laugh.

Complementary therapies

When people tell me they want to use complementary or alternative therapies, I always check out their belief in such remedies. I find that people quite often talk about a therapy and what they expect it to do – but rarely speak of their own role and what they can do to support the process. In other words, they are looking for the therapist to cure them. When using complementary therapies, I would encourage you to work *with* your therapist using your own thoughts and images.

One woman admitted that during her reflexology session she spent the time thinking about what she needed from the shops and suchlike, rather than what the therapist was doing or saying! I suggested that the therapy would be more effective if she used deep breathing techniques (see Chapter 5) and positive imagery (see Chapter 7) along with a simple relaxation routine. The outcome was that she felt more relaxed and, in her words, 'believing' in herself – in other words, she now believed more in her own ability to contribute to the healing process, rather than totally depending on the therapist.

This kind of proactive approach is invaluable in both orthodox or complementary medicine, instilling a belief that people can help to support such processes and ultimately themselves. So if you are trying these therapies, ensure you close your eyes and, if nothing else, imagine the fresh oxygen going to the area of the body that is being worked and helping it to heal.

15
A word about strokes

While most of this book relates to CHD, many people in my classes have also experienced strokes of varying intensity. All the factors already discussed are relevant for anyone who has suffered a stroke.

However, there are additional difficulties which slow down the recovery process, the main ones being frustration from the inability (either temporary or permanent) to think and talk clearly, or to control involuntary movement of limbs. As well as following the advice in this book, you might like to consider the additional factors in this chapter. If you have any points of concern, do consult your doctor.

Additional points for those who have had a stroke

Rehabilitation

This should start as soon after a stroke as possible. In your mind and in your actions, strive for independence, but also allow your family to support you; find solutions together.

Exercise

If you have a heart condition as well as a stroke, do join a rehab course. Initially progress may seem slow, but will soon improve.

Always consult your doctor before embarking on an exercise programme, and join a class with a professional tutor who understands your needs and capabilities. When using the exercise programmes as detailed in this book, always start with stage 1 and encourage a family member or friend to join in with you.

Try out all the sitting exercises in this book, but be careful with the standing ones, which require balance. You may need to wait a few months before you try these; consult your doctor.

A static exercise bike and swimming have both been of particular benefit to my stroke students, improving circulation and muscle strength.

An exercise training organization developed by a stroke survivor and a martial arts expert, called the ARNI Group (Action for Rehabilitation from Neurological Injury), provides trainers who work one-to-one with individuals to get back as much real function as possible (see Useful addresses).

Emotions

Have a look at the techniques for dealing with frustration in this book, especially the 'binning' technique (see page 27). Not being able to write clearly is very frustrating, but with perseverance it will improve; alternatively, as one of my students has found with great success, you can learn to write with your other hand.

Tiredness

Your condition will affect your alertness and create frequent bouts of loss of concentration, tiredness or fatigue. While it is important to be active, it is also important to rest. Do not fight tiredness; you will only feel more tired, often in the evening when tiredness can result in your speech beginning to slur. Taking a deep breath before speaking has helped all the students in my class.

Physical symptoms

Spasticity in the affected arm and leg that is tightening in the bent position can be brought on by effort, anxiety or fatigue and is often worse at the end of the day. To some extent this is preventable by good positioning of the arm or leg and also recognizing symptoms whereby the limb is ready to go into spasm, and managing to stop it. A physiotherapist will be able to advise you how to use this technique.

Over time, all my stroke students showed improvement in speech and also mobility in the limbs affected by their stroke. For example, Den said, 'I admit it did not seem possible, considering the state I was in when I first joined six months ago, that I would feel the benefits that I do now.'

A very good booklet, *Recovery from a Stroke*, is available free from the British Heart Foundation. Two other excellent booklets are available to help families give support and assist in the recovery period after a stroke: *Home Care for Patients in the Early Days* and *Understanding Stroke Illness*. Both are obtainable from the Chest, Heart and Stroke Foundation (see Useful addresses).

16

Week-by-week programme of recovery

This chapter contains progressive programmes of 'safe' guidelines to support your recovery. But they are just that, guidelines, dependent on the severity of your illness and your level of fitness before your illness was diagnosed. Those who have had surgery would benefit from following the complete programme. However, even if you have a condition that does not require surgery, the heart has had a shock. Give it, and yourself, time to rest. Err on the side of caution and your body will naturally progress to a level of competence and improved health. And, if you are concerned about the pace of your recovery, consult your doctor.

Weeks 1 and 2

Trying to make immediate change can feel like a punishment and make recovery more difficult. Take things easy for the first few days and acclimatize yourself to your surroundings.

Allow yourself a lie-in in the morning, but never stay in bed all day unless you have been medically advised to do so. Have loose cool clothing ready to put on (several layers) and, if necessary, allow others to help you. Take your time, breathe through each movement.

Take frequent rests – lying on your bed is best (at least twice a day). If lying down or getting up is difficult, read my guidelines on page 47. If you have difficulty sleeping at night, read pages 21–23.

Eat well, but have small meals up to six times a day. Make three of these fruit snacks. Always eat at the table, as your posture is better. After eating, sit for at least 10 minutes to help digestion. Do not read or watch television while you eat.

Drink plenty of water during the day – have a glass of water between hot drinks, and do not drink alcohol for the first two weeks.

Read through the advice sheets you brought home from hospital and read Chapter 2 of this book.

Share any 'down' feelings either by 'binning' (page 27) or by talking to your coronary care nurse, doctor, friends or family.

Only see visitors at your best time of day, and only for an hour at a time. Ask them not to visit if they have a cold or infection of any kind.

Read through the sections in this book. Take your time, and discuss things with your carer. Write a list of the changes you would like to make in your life, but don't act upon them yet.

Visit your doctor and pass on your discharge letter; let him/her know how you are feeling, and ensure you get any necessary medication. Have your medicine container ready and filled with your week's medicines. Aim to take them at the same time every day (see pages 15–16).

Good posture will help you to recover better – re-read page 50. Make a note in your 'Coaching Myself to Health Book' of your level of fitness since your illness was first diagnosed, and at the end of each two-week period grade yourself from 1 to 10.

Practise the circulation exercises and breathing exercises while sitting down (pages 106–7). Practise simple walking exercises in the home (pages 110–111).

Try not to watch television all day. Read, do quizzes or games or just listen to music.

If it is a pleasant day, aim to sit outside for at least an hour (dress appropriately for the weather).

Make notes during the weeks of any physical aspects of your recovery that are concerning you. If they are not major concerns, keep them for your outpatients appointment. If they are causing concern, immediately book an appointment with your GP or go to Accident & Emergency at your local hospital.

I doubt many of you will feel like smoking at this time, but if you are still a smoker, please read Chapter 9 and choose one of the 'giving up' strategies.

Weeks 3 and 4

Some of you will be feeling considerably better by now, but others will still be feeling weak. For the latter, continue with the programme as for weeks 1 and 2. For those who feel ready to do more, add in the following:

Reduce your rest periods, but have at least one nap a day as well as your night's sleep.

Keep up the circulation, breathing and the hourly going upstairs exercises. Start practising the warm-up exercises while sitting down (pages 108–110).

Read the section on healing imagery (pages 61–3) and choose an image to help your body to heal. Use this image with the basic relaxation script (page 130).

Review the information you have on healthy eating, and discuss with others what changes you want and need to make. Write a list in your 'Coaching Myself to Health Book' and make a note at the end of each week as to how you feel such changes are affecting you. Choose two dietary change aspects, and alter one a week.

Start the daily 'walking outside' programme beginning with Walk 1 (page 122). If you have not had surgery, you can safely begin Walk 2. Continue every day for two weeks.

If you are still feeling down, re-read pages 4 and 5 and Chapter 3.

Every time you feel frustrated or stressed, re-read Chapter 4.

Weeks 5 and 6

By now, most of you will be feeling stronger and ready to progress; if not, just repeat weeks 3 and 4.

Continue with all the warm-up exercises while sitting down and begin to incorporate the standing warm-up exercises (pages 111–120).

Continue to use the healing and relaxation imagery.

Implement two new dietary aims and, if you wish, include a couple of alcoholic drinks a week.

You may still be experiencing emotional ups and downs. This is quite normal – re-read Chapter 3.

Continue the daily walking programme by progressing to Walk 2 (page 122) or, if you began with Walk 2, progress to Walk 3. Ensure you use the breathing technique and dress appropriately for the weather (page 51).

Listen to a relaxation tape or practise the relaxation routine (see Chapter 14).

Start to make out a prioritizing list of things that you would like to do, and aim for one task to be completed a day (one that should not take longer than 30 minutes to complete; see page 69).

The outpatients appointment is usually at this time. Ensure you have your list of questions ready, plus any side effects of medication or difficulties experienced since you last saw the consultant (see page 17). If you wish to drive again or return to work, ensure these questions are on the list.

If you are able to return to work, make sure you read pages 10–11.

Put away any money you save from not smoking and reward yourself with a break away from home.

Check out your nearest heart support group and go along to meet everyone. The BHF has details of local contacts (see Useful addresses).

Weeks 7 and 8

Rest in the afternoons, even if you do not need to nap; just relax, listen to music or a relaxation tape.

Most people can start driving again, but for some the chest scar is still sore or they feel anxious. Read the coping guidelines on pages 8 and 48–9.

Choose two more dietary changes and implement one a week.

Allow yourself to prioritize one task a day, one that can take up to an hour to complete.

Maintain your circulatory and exercise routines and increase your walking programme by one number, which means you will now have progressed to either Walk 3 (30 minutes' duration) or Walk 4 (40 minutes' duration).

Continue to use the relaxation and imagery healing scripts.

Weeks 9 and 10

Rest in the afternoons; even if you do not need to nap, just relax, and listen to music or a relaxation tape.

Choose two more dietary changes and implement one a week.

Remember to make a note of how you feel at the end of each week.

Allow yourself to prioritize two tasks a day, which can take up to an hour each to complete – one in the morning, one in the afternoon.

Maintain your circulatory and exercise routines and increase your walking programme by one number, which means you will now have progressed to either Walk 4 (40 minutes' duration) or Walk 5 (60 minutes' duration). However, if this is still too much for you, stay with the programme that makes you feel a little tired but not breathless.

Continue to use the relaxation and imagery healing scripts.

Maintain your non-smoking regime if you have been following one; and if you have been, or still are, a heavy drinker, cut down.

Weeks 11 and 12

How are you feeling now? If you are following this programme carefully, I believe you will be feeling much better; for many, you will be feeling even stronger than you did before your illness was diagnosed. This is the time to look again at your list of desired lifestyle changes and evaluate how well you have done. Are there any that have not shown any improvement? If so, re-read the relevant chapters and start again. Although this is review time, it does not mean you can rest on your laurels and not bother to seek further change. In fact, I expect you to be motivated to continue! Let all the processes we have discussed become second nature, and continue with the following:

- Daily circulatory exercises while sitting down.
- Daily warm-up sitting and standing exercises.
- Daily walking programme.
- Breathing techniques done frequently throughout the day.
- Challenging any *health-inhibiting thoughts (hits)* and replacing with *health-enhancing practices (heps)*.
- Using your healing imagery until you feel your body has sufficiently recovered.

Also consider:

- Buying an exercise bike and using it at home.
- Joining a coronary exercise class or a gym that specializes in working with people with coronary heart disease.
- Rewarding yourself and your carer with a break away. It is probably best to start in this country, and somewhere fairly close to home, peaceful and relaxing. Plan it yourself: find out the distances and terrain of various nature trails and walks where you can enjoy the scenery and keep up your active walking programme. Remember the timing needs to include the return jour-

ney. Make sure you take adequate supplies of your required medication and know where the nearest doctor or hospital is.

After six months

By now you should have experienced great change and an increased sense of well-being, so exercise programmes can be adapted to suit your lifestyle. However, you should exercise for at least one hour every other day.

After one year

Anniversaries are often milestones. This is a time of reflection, sometimes rekindled fear, but most importantly it is a time of recognition of how far you have come. Read through your self-help health booklet and note any changes, then put it away for safe keeping and only refer to it again if the need arises.

For ever...

I know so many people, all of whom have suffered as you have, many over 20 years ago. How well they are now! They have a message for you: 'Although it was hard at times, we did it –and so can you!'

Useful addresses

For rehabilitation classes or voice tapes, email iatubbs@aol.com. Or visit optimumwellbeing.org.uk

Alcohol

Addiction Network
Website: www.addictionnetwork.co.uk
Email: hello@addictionnetwork.co.uk

A site to help people with drinking and drug-addiction problems.

Alcoholics Anonymous
PO Box 1
Stonebow House
Stonebow
York YO1 7NJ
Tel.: 01904 644026
Response line: 0800 55 7 4 55
Website: alcoholicsanonymous.org.uk
www.al-anonuk.org.uk (for families)

Alcohol Concern
Waterbridge House
32–36 Loman Street
London SE1 0EE
Tel.: 020 7928 7377
Website: www.alcoholconcern.org.uk
Email: contact@alcoholconcern.org.uk

Drinkline 0800 917 82 82

KCA (UK) Drugs and Alcohol Service
Dan House
44 East Street
Faversham
Kent ME13 8AT
Tel.: 01795 590635
Website: www.kca.org.uk
Email: admin@kca.org.uk

Provides a range of community services in various bases across Kent for individuals affected by alcohol or drug misuse.

Portman Group
Tel.: 020 7907 3700

A helpline established by the drinks industry to promote responsible drinking and to foster a balanced understanding of alcohol-related issues. Best time to phone: Monday to Friday 9 am to 5 pm.

Sober Recovery
www.soberrecovery.com
International site includes a directory containing hundreds of drug rehabilitation and addiction treatment centres worldwide.

Complementary Medicine

British Medical Acupuncture Society (BMAS)
BMAS House
3 Winnington Court
Northwich
Cheshire CW8 1AQ
Tel.: 01606 786782
Website: www.medical-acupuncture.co.uk
Email: admin@medical-acupuncture.org.uk

General Council for Massage Therapy
Whiteway House
Blundells Lane
Rainhill
Prescot
L35 6NB
Tel.: 0870 850 4452
Website: www.gcmt.org.uk
Email: gcmt@btconnect.com

Institute of Complementary Medicine (ICM)
PO Box 194
London SE16 7QZ
Tel.: 020 7237 5165 between 10 am and 12.30 pm or write for list of practitioners to the Information Officer, enclosing s.a.e.
Website: www.i-c-m.org.uk
Email info@i-c-m.org.uk

International Register of Consultant Herbalists and Homoeopaths
32 King Edward Road
Swansea
SA1 4LL
Tel.: 01792 655 886
Website: www.irch.org
Email: office@irch.org

Coronary Heart Disease and Stroke

Action for Rehabilitation from Neurological Injury (ARNI)
PO Box 68
Lingfield
Surrey
RH7 6QQ

British Cardiac Patients Association (BCPA)
National Helpline 01223 846845
Website: www.bcpa.co.uk
Email (for assistance): HelpMe@bcpa.co.uk

British Heart Foundation
14 Fitzhardinge Street
London W1H 6DH
Tel.: 020 7935 0185
Heart info line: 08450 70 80 70, Monday to Friday, 9 am to 5 pm: free service for those seeking information on heart health issues.
Website: www.bhf.org.uk
BHF statistics website: www.heartstats.org
Email: internet@bhf.org.uk

BHF also produces various booklets and resources, and these are available to download from the website or order from there by emailing orderline@bhf.org.uk

British Hypertension Society
Website: www.bhsoc.org.uk

Countryside Commission
Walking for Health promotion
John Dower House
Crescent Place
Cheltenham
Gloucestershire
GL50 3RA
Tel.: 01242 521381

Department of Health
0800 555777 (literature line); 08701 555455 (response line)

The Department of Health and the Department for Education and Skills have developed a series of websites to provide information for a range of audiences that relates to the National Curriculum and the National Healthy Schools Programme. See www.wiredforhealth.gov.uk

Family Heart Association ***see*** **H E A R T UK**

H E A R T UK
7 North Road
Maidenhead
Berkshire
SL6 1PE

Tel.: 01628 628638
Website: www.heartuk.org.uk
Email:ask@heartuk.org.uk

Stroke Association
Stroke Information Service
The Stroke Association
240 City Road
London EC1V 2AL
Helpline: 0845 3033 100, Monday to Friday, 9 am to 5 pm
Website: www.stroke.org.uk
Email: info@stroke.org.uk

Counselling

British Association of Behavioural and Cognitive Psychotherapies (BABCP)
The Globe Centre
PO Box 9
Accrington
Lancashire BB5 0XB
Tel.: 01254 875277
Website: www.babcp.org.uk
Email: babcp@babcp.com

British Association for Counselling and Psychotherapy
BACP House
35–37 Albert Street
Rugby
Warwickshire
CV21 2SG
Tel.: 0870 443 5252
Website: www.bacp.co.uk
Email: bacp@bacp.co.uk

Disseminates counselling and psychotherapy information to the public.

Carers UK
20–25 Glasshouse Yard
London EC1A 4JT
CarersLine 0808 808 7777 Wednesdays/Thursdays 10 am to 12 pm/ 2–4 pm
Website: www.carersuk.org
Email info@carersuk.org

All aspects of caring; the voice of carers and the only carer-led organization working for all carers.

Institute of Psychosexual Medicine
12 Chandos Street
Cavendish Square
London W1G 9DR
Tel.: 020 7580 0631
Website: www.ipm.org.uk

To contact the Institute, write in first instance including s.a.e. to receive a list of doctors in your local area trained to help with sexual problems following heart surgery.

International Stress Management Association UK (ISMA UK)
PO Box 26
South Petherton
TA13 5WY
Tel. 07000 780430
Website: www.isma.org.uk
Email: stress@isma.org.uk

No Panic (National Association for Phobias, Anxiety, Neuroses, Information and Care)
93 Brands Farm Way
Randlay
Telford
Shropshire TF3 2JQ
Helpline (freephone) 0808 808 0545 (10 am to 10 pm daily)
Tel. (admin): 01952 590 005 (office hours)
Website: www.nopanic.co.uk

Relate
Central Office
Herbert Gray College
Little Church Street
Rugby
Warwickshire CV21 3AP
Tel.: 0845 456 1310
Website: relate.org.uk
Email: enquiries@ relate.org.uk

The Sexual Dysfunction Association
Windmill Place Business Centre
2–4 Windmill Lane
Southall
Middlesex UB2 4NJ
Tel.: 0870 774 3571
Website: sda.uk.net
Email: info@sda.uk.net

Westminster Pastoral Foundation (for WPF counselling)
23 Kensington Square
London W8 5HN
Tel.: 020 7361 4803/4
Website: www.wpf.org.uk
Email: counselling@wpf.org.uk

Smoking

Action on Smoking and Health (ASH)
Website: www.ash.org.uk

NHS Smoking Helpline 0800 169 0 169 (UK)

A 90-day programme to stop smoking can be found on www.netdoctor.co.uk
Another helpful website is www.givingupsmoking.co.uk

Quitline (to aid giving up smoking)
0800 00 22 00 (UK)
Website: www.quit.org.uk
Email: stopsmoking@quit.org.uk
Website: sda.co.uk
Email: info@sda.uk.net

Smokeline (Scotland)
0800 84 84 84

Smokeline (Wales)
0800 169 0 169 (bilingual). Lines open Tuesdays 12 noon to midnight

Smokers Quitline (Northern Ireland)
0800 848 484. Lines open Tuesdays 12 noon to midnight

General

Age Concern
Freephone helpline 0800 00 99 66, 8 am to 7 pm, 7 days a week
Website: www.ageconcern.org.uk

British Dental Health Foundation
Helpline 0870 333 1188
Website: www.dentalhealth.org.uk

British Nutrition Foundation
Tel.: 020 7404 6504
Website: www.nutrition.org.uk

Driving and Vehicle Licensing Agency (DVLA)
Helpline 0870 600 0301, Mondays to Fridays, 8.15 am to 4.30 pm
(for enquiries about driving and medical conditions)
Website: www.dvla.gov.uk

Further Reading

An extensive range of books is available from the British Heart Foundation. See under Useful addresses.

American Heart Association, *No-Fad Diet: A Personal Plan for Healthy Weight Loss*. Clarkson N. Potter, New York, 2005.

Brown, Lynda, *The Insomniac's Best Friend*. HarperCollins, London, 2004.

Burkman, Kip, *The Stroke Recovery Book: A Guide for Patients and Families*. Addicus Books, Omaha, Nebr., 1998, rev. edn 2005.

Burns, David, *The Feeling Good Handbook*. Plume, New York, 1990.

Butler, Gillian, and Hope, Tony, *Manage Your Mind: The Mental Fitness Guide*. Oxford Paperbacks, Oxford, 1995.

Carr, Allen, *Packing it in the Easy Way*. Available from the author on 0800 3892115; www.allencarreasyway.com

Chaitow, Leon, *The Stress Protection Plan*. Thorsons, London, 1992.

Cleland, John, *Understanding Heart Failure*. Family Doctor Publications Ltd, Poole, 2003.

Cornel, Chin, *Exercise for Everyone*. Quadrille Publishing, London, 2004.

Dyke, Pat and Dyke, Colin, *Relaxation in a Week*. Hodder & Stoughton, London, 1992.

France, Christine, *Low Cholesterol, Low Fat; Recipes for a Healthy Heart*. Southwater, London, 2000.

Hewitt, James, *The Complete Relaxation Book*. Rider, London, 1989.

Houghton, Andrew R. and Gray, David, *Making Sense of the ECG*. Hodder Arnold, London, 2003.

Kowalski, Robert, *The New 8-Week Cholesterol Cure: The Ultimate Program for Preventing Heart Disease*. HarperCollins, New York, 2003.

Lilly, Leonard (ed.), *Pathophysiology of Heart Disease*. Lippincott Williams and Wilkins, London, 2002.

Lindenfield, Gael, *Assert Yourself*. Thorsons/Element, London, new edn 2004.

Lynas, Jacquie, *Cooking for a Healthy Heart*. Hamlyn, London, 2004.

Madders, James, *The Stress and Relaxation Handbook*. Vermilion, London, second edn 1997.

Madders, Jane, *Relax and Be Happy*. Unwin, London, 1987.

Mitchell, Laura, *Simple Relaxation*. John Murray, London, 1988.

Newby, David, et al., *Coronary Heart Disease: Your Questions Answered*. Churchill Livingstone, London, 2004.

Opie, Lionel, *Drugs for the Heart*. W. B. Saunders Ltd, London, 2004.

Palmer, Stephen et al. *Creating a Balance: Managing Stress*. British Library Publishing Division, London, 2003.

Proto, L. *Total Relaxation in Five Steps*. London, Penguin, 1991.

Rowlands, Barbara, *The Which? Guide to Complementary Medicine*. Which? Ltd, London, 1997.

Shreeve, Caroline, *How to Lower High Blood Pressure: The Natural Four Point Plan to Reduce Hypertension*. HarperCollins, London, 2001.

Talbott, Shawn, *The Cortisol Connection: Why Stress Makes You Fat and Ruins Your Health and What You Can do About It*. Hunter House, Alameda, Calif., 2002.

Tallis, Frank, *How to Stop Worrying*. Sheldon Press (Overcoming Common Problems Series), London, 1990.

Tubbs, Irene, *Creative Relaxation in Groupwork*. Speechmark Publishing, Bicester, 1996.

Index